ARTHRITIS
AND INFLAMMATION

NOTE

This publication was written by registered dietitians to provide insights into better eating habits to promote health and wellness. It does not provide a cure for any specific ailment or condition and is not a substitute for the advice and/or treatment given by a licensed physician.

First published in French in 2013 by Les Publications Modus Vivendi Inc. under the title *Arthrite et inflammation*.
© Elisabeth Cerqueira, Marise Charron and Les Publications Modus Vivendi Inc., 2016

MODUS VIVENDI PUBLISHING

55 Jean-Talon Street West
Montreal, Quebec H2R 2W8
CANADA

modusvivendipublishing.com

Publisher: Marc G. Alain
Editorial director: Isabelle Jodoin
Editorial assistant and copy editor: Nolwenn Gouezel
English-language editor: Carol Sherman
Translator: Rhonda Mullins
Proofreader: Maeve Haldane
Graphic designers: Émilie Houle and Gabrielle Lecomte
Food photographer: André Noël
Food stylist: Gabrielle Dalessandro
Authors' photographer: OVATIO.ca
Additional photography:
Pages 5, 6, 12, 16, 19, 23, 24, 26, 28, 33, 38 to 47, 49 to 52, 55, 56, 62, 67, 70, 80
82, 86, 98, 101, 104, 111, 134, 154, 157 and 158: Dreamstime.com
Pages 76, 89, 130 and 132: Stockxchng.com
Pages 21, 38, 39, 45, 48, 51 and 55: iStock

ISBN: 978-1-77286-008-5 (PAPERBACK)

ISBN: 978-1-77286-009-2 (PDF)
ISBN: 978-1-77286-010-8 (EPUB)
ISBN: 978-1-77286-011-5 (KINDLE)

Legal deposit – Bibliothèque et Archives nationales du Québec, 2016
Legal deposit – Library and Archives Canada, 2016

We gratefully acknowledge the financial support of the Government of Canada through the Canada Book Fund (CBF) for our publishing activities.

Government of Quebec – Tax Credit for Book Publishing – Program administered by SODEC

Printed in Canada

KNOW WHAT TO EAT

ARTHRITIS AND INFLAMMATION

21 DAYS OF MENUS

Elisabeth Cerqueira and Marise Charron, RD

MODUS VIVENDI

CONTENTS

INTRODUCTION 7

ARTHRITIS 8

Biology 101 8

The Probable Causes of Arthritis 10

Watching Your Waistline and BMI 10

DAILY DIETARY RECOMMENDATIONS 13

Choose an Anti-inflammatory Diet 14

Stay Hydrated 17

Eat Plenty of Fiber 18

Consume More Antioxidants and Phytonutrients 20

Choose Omega-3s Over Omega-6s 22

Eat a Mediterranean Diet 24

Strengthen Your Intestinal Wall 25

Identify Allergies and Food Intolerances 26

Avoid Proinflammatory Fats 27

Reduce Your Intake of Refined Sugar 29

Foods to Choose 30

Foods to Avoid 31

Food Recommendations for Gout 32

21 DAYS OF MENUS 35

RECIPES - 47 HEALTHY IDEAS **59**

Drinks 60

Breakfast and Sweet Snacks 68

Appetizers, Sides and Savory Snacks 76

Soups and Salads 86

Main Courses 111

Desserts 144

ABOUT THE AUTHORS **153**

ACKNOWLEDGMENTS **155**

RESOURCES FOR ARTHRITIS SUFFERERS **156**

RECIPE INDEX **159**

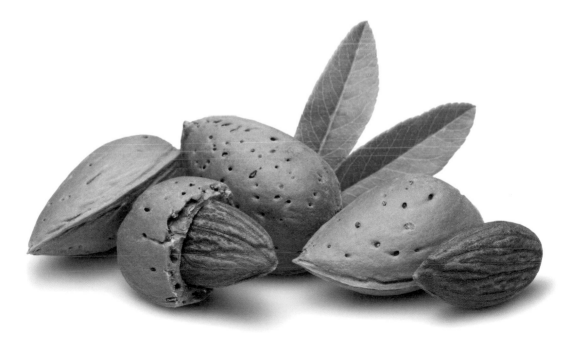

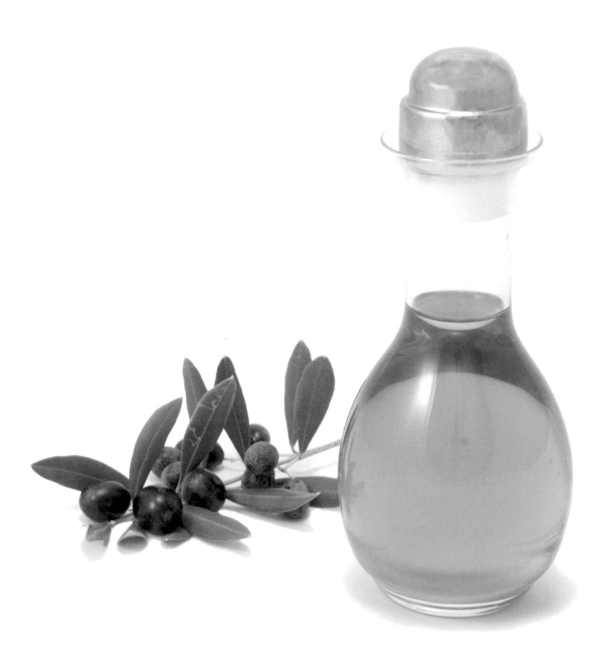

INTRODUCTION

Arthritis (from the Greek *arthro*, which means "joint," and *itis*, which means "inflammation") is an inflammation of one or more joints (knees, hands, feet, hips, spine, etc.). The disease can affect cartilage, ligaments, tendons or any other part of the musculoskeletal system.

Arthritis is an autoimmune disease in which the immune system attacks the joints. It's a bit like a general ordering his troops to fire on their own side rather than on the enemy. The result is chronic inflammation of the mucous membrane of the joints, particularly in the hands and feet (rheumatoid arthritis). The inflammation can spread to other tissue surrounding the joints. Arthritis is a progressive disease that often results in deformed joints and, ultimately, disability.

While arthritis is a lifelong affliction, the symptoms can fluctuate over time. When symptoms are present, the disease is said to be "active"; the patient suffers from muscle and joint pain, and joints are red and swollen.

Arthritis affects women in particular, but the causes are still unknown, and onset can occur at any age. There is no known cure. However, there is a range of medication, targeted exercises and techniques to protect the joints that can help manage arthritis. Fortunately, many scientific studies have demonstrated the role of diet in preventing the progression of the disease and reducing inflammation. The nutritional advice offered here may help control symptoms.

ARTHRITIS

BIOLOGY 101

A joint is the connection between two bones, which are protected at either end by cartilage that act as a cushion between the joints. The synovial cavity is found between two areas of cartilage that come into contact. It contains a lubricant that enables fluid, pain-free movement. When there is a reduction in cartilage or synovial fluid, inflammation and swelling of the joints can result, which can be painful. Over time, the cartilage can crack and disappear altogether, leaving the bone exposed.

There are two major categories of arthritis: rheumatoid arthritis and related diseases (juvenile arthritis, ankylosing spondylitis, psoriatic arthritis and gout), and osteoarthritis. The common denominator in all forms of arthritis is joint and musculoskeletal pain.

Rheumatoid arthritis refers to an inflammation of the joint capsule's mucous membrane (the synovial membrane). Initially, the affected joints are swollen, painful and warm and sensitive to the touch. Gradually as the disease progresses, the synovial membrane releases enzymes into the joint that can dissolve the bone and the cartilage. At this stage, the joint can become deformed, and the pain becomes unbearable. It is not known what triggers rheumatoid arthritis, or what causes it to go into remission or brings on an attack.

Inflammatory forms of arthritis are related to an immune system dysfunction. Antibodies attack the joint membranes and can attack other organs such as the eyes, lungs and heart.

Gout is a particular form of arthritis. It affects just under 2% of the population, particularly men. Gout causes episodes of pain in one or more joints. Any joint can be affected, but most often it is the big toe joint. The affected joint becomes purplish red and swollen.

An abnormally high level of uric acid in the blood is the cause of gout, which results from inadequate elimination of the acid in urine or increased synthesis of purines, its precursors. Uric acid is metabolic waste normally found in the body, but when there is too much of it (hyperuricemia), it settles drop by drop to form crystals, particularly around the joints. These deposits trigger inflammatory responses.

As for osteoarthritis, it is caused by the disintegration of the tissue that covers and protects the ends of the bones. The bones start to rub against each other, resulting in dysfunction, loss of mobility in the joint and pain.

As mentioned earlier, the common denominator in all those forms of arthritis is joint and musculoskeletal pain. Here are some of the other common symptoms:

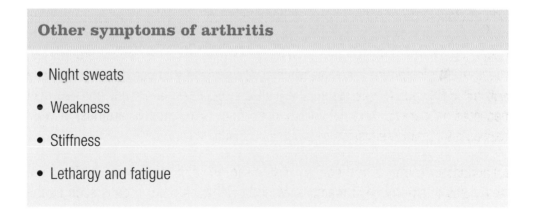

Other symptoms of arthritis

- Night sweats

- Weakness

- Stiffness

- Lethargy and fatigue

In cases of chronic pain, it is important to consult a doctor for a clear, accurate diagnosis and to find out about possible treatments.

THE PROBABLE CAUSES OF ARTHRITIS

Arthritis is a multifactor disorder. The following table summarizes the modifiable and non-modifiable causes.

Modifiable	Non-modifiable
• Diet	• Aging
• Sedentary lifestyle	• Sex (more prevalent among women)
• Alcohol intake	• Hormones
• Excess weight and obesity	• Genetic predisposition
• Joint trauma	
• Smoking	
• Viral infections	
• Working as a physical laborer	
• Past injuries	
• Weakened immune system	
• Intestinal permeability (a theory)	

WATCHING YOUR WAISTLINE AND BMI

Reducing your waistline and maintaining a healthy weight through a balanced diet and regular physical exercise are important factors in managing the disease.

Waistline	Men	Women
Ideal waistline	< 37 inches (94 cm)	< 32 inches (80 cm)
At-risk* waistline	> 40 inches (102 cm)	> 35 inches (88 cm)

* Waistline at which the risk of developing health problems is high (diabetes, cholesterol, high blood pressure, cancer, liver problems, etc.).

Calculating your BMI:

Your weight in pounds ÷ 2.2 = _____ kilograms

Your height (in meters) x your height (in meters) = _____ m²

Your BMI = your weight (in kg) ÷ your height squared (in m²)

Category	BMI (kg/m²)	Risk
Underweight	Below 18.5	Increased risk
Normal weight	18.5 to 24.9	Less risk
Overweight	25 to 29.9	Increased risk
Obesity class I	30 to 34.9	High risk
Obesity class II	35 to 39.9	Very high risk
Obesity class III	40 or higher	Extremely high risk

Does not apply to children, athletes, pregnant women or people over 65.

Losing weight reduces stress on your joints. Losing even a little weight can considerably reduce pain.

Fatty tissue around the waist is metabolically active. This abdominal fat releases proinflammatory cytokines, increasing the risk of inflammation in the body. Being active and in good shape reduces the cells' production of inflammatory molecules.

In addition to a balanced diet, physical activity is important: yoga, Pilates, tai chi, abdominal exercises, stretching (daily if possible), resistance training with light weights or elastics, walking outdoors, taking deep breaths, etc.

During physical effort, the body secretes endorphins, which act as a pain reliever. Exercise also improves circulation and increases endurance, which helps improve cardiovascular health. Some studies show that improved blood circulation resulting from increased blood flow after exercise stimulates an anti-inflammatory response in the cells of the blood vessels and also helps maintain the health of arteries and joints.

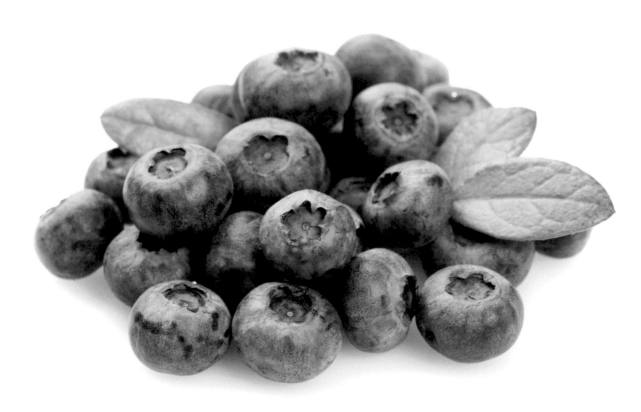

Recommendations

Adapting your diet to your health can be particularly beneficial for the body and can relieve certain symptoms. Here are some dietary recommendations to help you balance your diet and reduce pain related to inflammation.

You can also consult a dietitian for an anti-inflammatory dietary plan that reflects your tastes and the progression of the disease.

RECOMMENDATIONS:

1. Choose an anti-inflammatory diet
2. Drink plenty of fluids
3. Eat plenty of fiber
4. Consume antioxidants or phytonutrients
5. Choose omega-3s over omega 6s
6. Eat a Mediterranean diet
7. Strengthen your intestinal wall
8. Identify food allergies and intolerances
9. Avoid proinflammatory fats
10. Reduce your intake of refined sugar

1 CHOOSE AN ANTI-INFLAMMATORY DIET

To relieve arthritis pain, it is a good idea at every meal and at snack time to eat anti-inflammatory foods, tend toward a vegetarian diet and include more antioxidants.

FOODS WITH ANTI-INFLAMMATORY PROPERTIES

- **Fruits and vegetables**
  Fruits: apples, blueberries, cherries, kiwi, mango, papaya, peaches, pears, pineapple and strawberries.
  Vegetables: asparagus, avocado, broccoli, cabbage (green, kale or Brussels sprouts), celery, garlic, olives, onions, spinach, squash and sweet potato.

- **Fish and meat substitutes**
  Fish rich in omega-3s: herring, mackerel, salmon, sardines, trout and tuna.
  Legumes: chickpeas, all varieties of lentils and red beans.

- **Grains** (as unrefined and unprocessed as possible, consumed in their natural state)
  Buckwheat, millet, quinoa, brown rice and other whole-grain products.

- **Herbs and spices**
  Cilantro, turmeric, ginger, cinnamon, cumin and rosemary.

- **Nuts and seeds** (unsalted)
  Brazil nuts, almonds, sunflower seeds, ground flaxseeds, hemp seeds, chia seeds and pumpkin seeds. Try eating ¼ cup (60 ml) per day.

- **Certain oils**
  Extra virgin olive oil and coconut oil. (According to some studies, extra virgin olive oil could reduce inflammation similar to a non-steroid anti-inflammatory, such as ibuprofen or aspirin, because it contains oleocanthal, which blocks the enzymes that cause inflammation.)

TIPS FOR AN ANTI-INFLAMMATORY DIET

- Become a part-time vegetarian: for instance, try "meatless Mondays" and learn how to cook kale, which is rich in antioxidants.

- Eat berries (raspberries, blackberries, strawberries and blueberries) every day.

- Eat fatty fish two or three times a week and plan two to five or more meals with legumes weekly.

- Read labels and choose food with a short list of ingredients (a maximum of five).

- Cook with healthy fat and season dishes with herbs and spices.

- Prepare vinaigrettes with a healthy nut oil and apple cider vinegar.

- Aim for the healthy plate described below.

THE HEALTHY PLATE

Whether you are eating at home, a restaurant, a friend's house, a buffet or a cafeteria, follow the basic rule of the healthy plate to avoid making poor choices.

Half your plate should contain vegetables that are rich in antioxidants and anti-inflammatories; a quarter of the plate should contain grains (around the size of a fist); the other quarter should contain protein such as fish, lean white meat or legumes (around the size of the palm of your hand).

Get into the habit of serving yourself once and be aware of signals of hunger and fullness. Listen to your body, and your appetite!

For snacks, choose nuts, seeds, fruit or foods rich in calcium.

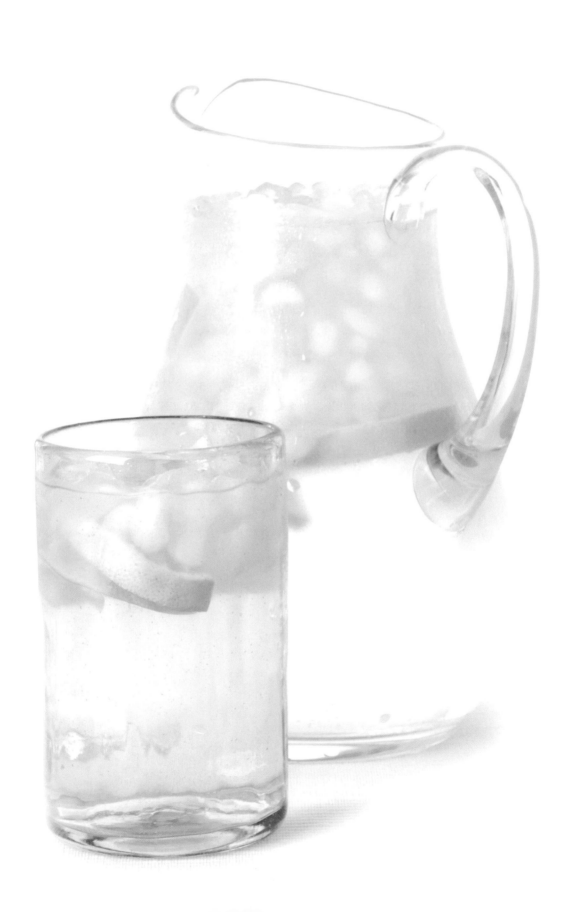

2 STAY HYDRATED

To lubricate your joints and relieve pain, you need to drink enough water every day, preferably filtered.

The Institute of Medicine determined that an adequate intake for men is about 13 cups (3.25 l) of total beverages a day. For women, it's about 9 cups (2.25 l) of total beverages a day.

Tips for staying hydrated

- To give water taste, add grated ginger, fresh mint, frozen berries, slices or zest of lemon or orange, or star anise.
- Make yourself some Anti-Inflammatory Water (see page 60).
- Drink green tea. The catechins found in green tea reduce inflammation and joint pain associated with rheumatoid arthritis. To get the most catechins, use leaf tea and steep for 5 minutes.

3 EAT PLENTY OF FIBER

Get all the benefits of fiber by including as many plant-based foods in your diet as possible. Fiber protects against cardiovascular disease, can prevent certain cancers and seems to reduce the level of C-reactive protein, an indicator of inflammation found in the blood. Be sure to eat at least 30 g of fiber every day.

Tips for increasing fiber in your diet

- Add chia seeds or flaxseeds to your menus.

- Use brown rice instead of white rice.

- Eat a variety of grains: millet, buckwheat, quinoa, amaranth and others.

- Eat more legumes.

- Aim for at least 2 cups (500 ml) of vegetables, preferably raw, and three servings of fresh fruit a day.

Don't forget to drink enough water to allow the fiber to do its work for intestinal health.

Recent studies show that a vegetarian or vegan diet significantly reduces symptoms and pain in people suffering from rheumatoid arthritis. So try including plenty of plant-based foods in your daily diet.

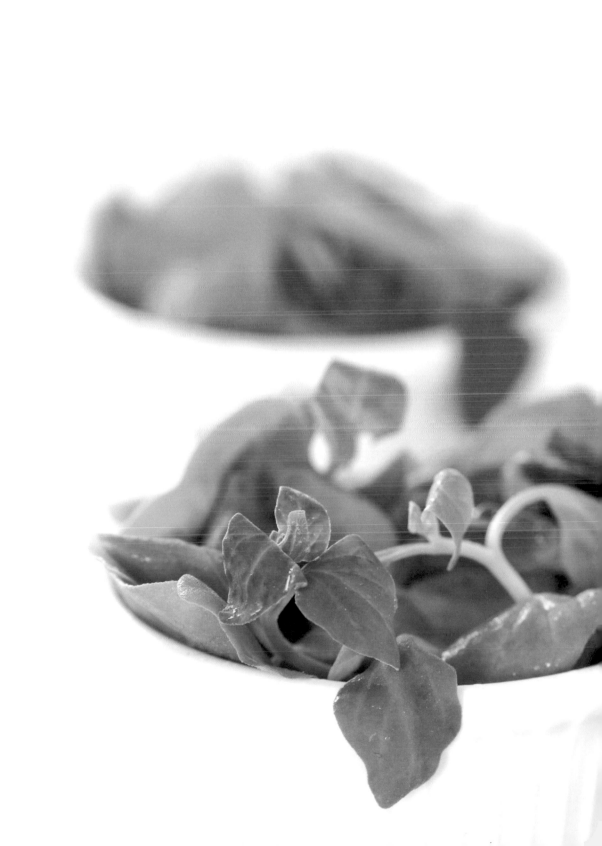

4 CONSUME MORE ANTIOXIDANTS AND PHYTONUTRIENTS

Antioxidants protect joints against the formation of free radicals that are partly responsible for inflammation. Studies show that certain antioxidants can help prevent arthritis, slow its progression and relieve pain.

Here are the ten best sources of antioxidants and anti-inflammatories. Try to consume at least five of the following ingredients every day.

- Anthocyanins: blackberries, black currants, blueberries, elderberries, cherries, raspberries, grapes (red, black or purple), strawberries, plums, cranberries, rhubarb, red wine, red onions and apples.

- Seasonings and spices: ginger, cayenne pepper and turmeric.

- Beta-carotene: sweet potatoes, carrots, kale, butternut squash, pumpkin, watermelon, apricots and spinach.

- Beta-cryptoxanthin: winter squash, pumpkin, persimmon, papaya, mandarins, oranges, apricots, carrots, nectarines and watermelon.

- Polyphenols and resveratrol: green tea and red wine, particularly Italian Cabernet Sauvignon, American Pinot Noir and Swiss Merlot.

- Quercetin: onions (red, yellow and white), kale, leeks, broccoli, blueberries, black currants, elderberries, cocoa powder (unsweetened), apricots, apples with the peel and black grapes.

- Vitamin C: citrus fruits, strawberries, kiwis, pineapple, kale, papaya, lemons, broccoli and Brussels sprouts.

- Vitamin D: wild salmon, mackerel, sardines, herring, egg yolks, mushrooms, enriched soy and almond milk.

- Vitamin E and omega-3s: fatty fish, chia seeds, hemp seeds, ground flaxseeds, nuts and wheat germ.

- Selenium: Brazil nuts (one Brazil nut daily meets your needs for selenium), canned light tuna (in water), crab, oysters, tilapia, cod, shrimp, wheat germ and whole-grain foods.

Tips for consuming more antioxidants and phytonutrients

- Eat one or two Brazil nuts and a small handful of walnuts every day.

- Add ground flaxseeds to your cereal, soup, yogurt and salads.

- Eat more meat substitutes and fish rich in omega-3s.

- Season dishes with herbs and spices.

- Eat 2 cups (500 ml) of vegetables and fruit rich in vitamin C daily (citrus fruit, pineapple).

- Drink green tea every day.

We recommend changing your diet rather than using supplements. Before taking supplements, it is strongly recommended that you talk to your doctor and your dietician to avoid interactions with your medication or overdose.

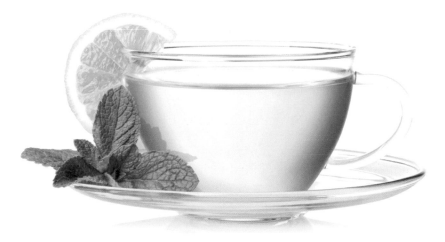

5 CHOOSE OMEGA-3S OVER OMEGA-6S

Omega-3 fatty acids are healthy fats for people suffering from arthritis. A diet rich in omega-3s, associated in some cases with fish oil as a supplement, may be recommended for those suffering from arthritis.

To reduce joint inflammation, it is a good idea to increase your consumption of foods rich in omega-3s (marine sources are best) and reduce your consumption of foods rich in omega-6s.

Foods rich in omega-3s to eat more of:

- Fatty fish: salmon (wild, fresh or canned), herring, mackerel, sardines, anchovies
- Chia seeds, ground flaxseeds, pumpkin seeds, hemp seeds
- Walnuts
- Nut oils
- Algae

Foods rich in omega-6s to avoid:

- Soybean, corn and sunflower oils
- Offal (liver, kidneys)
- Fatty meats
- Commercial pastry with hydrogenated oils
- Processed foods with hydrogenated oils

Clinical trials with fish oil supplements have shown that high doses, i.e. 500 to 1000 mg per capsule, of these supplements (EPA and DHA) may reduce symptoms of rheumatoid arthritis, such as how long morning stiffness lasts, the number of swollen, sensitive joints and pain. It can take up to three month to relieve symptoms.

Reducing the consumption of omega-6 polyunsaturated fatty acids in your diet while taking these supplements can make treatment more effective. Be careful: fish oil can interact with certain medications. Always ask your doctor's advice.

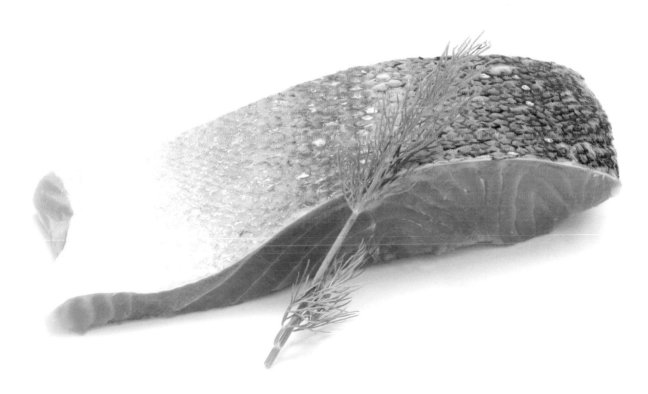

6 EAT A MEDITERRANEAN DIET

A study was conducted among Swedes suffering from polyarthritis (a condition that involves five or more joints). Significant relief of symptoms was observed among participants who adopted a Mediterranean diet for three months: reduced pain and inflammation and significant drop in the disease's activity and the number of swollen joints. However, studies are ongoing to determine the long-term effects of this diet.

The main ingredients in the Mediterranean diet are fatty fish, nuts and olive oil. Fresh fruit and vegetables consumed in large quantities and red wine consumed in moderation produce a range of antioxidants that protect against proinflammatory cytokines and free radicals involved in the inflammation process. Red meat is consumed in moderation.

People who live in the Mediterranean basin enjoy the fresh air and keep stress to a minimum, factors that may also promote their general well being.

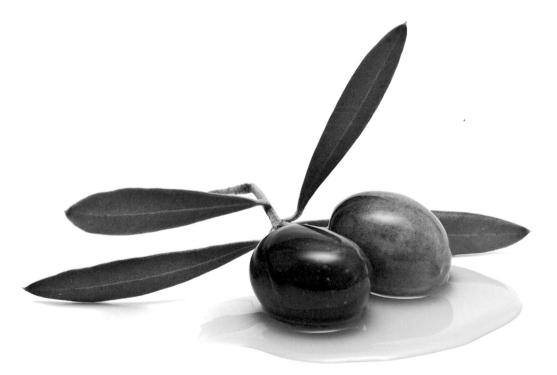

7 STRENGTHEN YOUR INTESTINAL WALL

The intestinal wall is the digestive system's first line of defense. Sometimes (with illness, infections and stress), this barrier can become permeable and let unwanted substances through. Substances that normally don't pass through this barrier or that do so in a limited way may harm your health and your body.

Diet can be a simple, inexpensive way to restore the barrier's effectiveness and strengthen your digestive system. Substances that offer potential for this include glutamine, probiotics, foods rich in enzymes, fiber and turmeric.

If you suffer from constipation, diarrhea, bloating or gas, it is important to treat these problems and work toward optimal intestinal health.

Tips for improving intestinal health

- Choose foods rich in glutamine (spinach, legumes, fish, parsley, miso and others).

- Consume probiotics to maintain optimal intestinal flora.

- Eat raw foods rich in enzymes: fruits (papaya, pineapple, kiwi and others), nuts, raw vegetables, sprouts and fresh herbs

- Choose food rich in dietary fiber, preferably whole grains.

- Each foods rich in omega-3s.

- Add turmeric to your favorite foods.

- Drink at least 8 cups (2 l) of water a day.

8 IDENTIFY ALLERGIES AND FOOD INTOLERANCES

A food journal is the best way to find out whether you have any food intolerances. You should note what you eat at every meal and identify associated symptoms. If you have doubts about a particular food, eliminate it from your diet and see if you feel better. Reintegrate the food later to see if the symptoms reappear. Listen to your body.

If you want to try a hypoallergenic diet, be sure you are working with a dietitian to avoid creating dietary deficiencies, which can arise when you eliminate dairy products, meat or wheat.

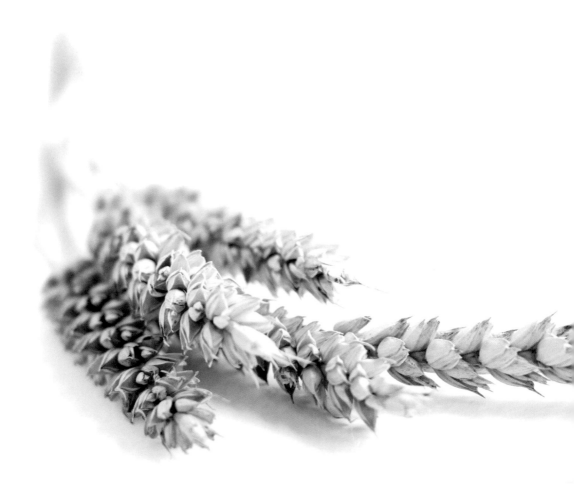

7 AVOID PROINFLAMMATORY FATS

These are mainly saturated and hydrogenated fats.

Saturated fats

20% m.f. cheese, cream, butter, fatty meats and cold cuts

Hydrogenated fats

Essentially palm oil (contained in crackers, cookies, granola bars and any other packaged baked goods)

Limit your consumption of saturated fats by choosing cheese with less than 20% m.f. and dairy products with 2% m.f. or less. Choose enriched plant-based milk (soy, almond, rice and others) and lean poultry. Cook at a low temperature.

To avoid hydrogenated fats, choose homemade bars, cookies and pastries over commercial products.

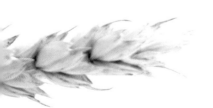

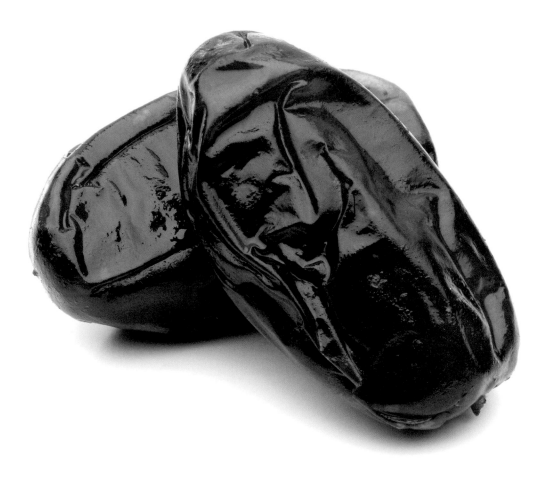

10 REDUCE YOUR INTAKE OF REFINED SUGAR

Consumed in large quantities, refined sugars (see the following list) aggravate arthritis pain by promoting inflammation.

- Granulated sugar and brown sugar

- Soft drinks and fruit punch

- Refined cereals, granola bars, cookies, pastries

- Chocolate (less than 70% cocoa)

Tips for reducing the amount of refined sugar in your diet

- Avoid or limit your consumption of food with simple, refined carbohydrates (refined enriched flour, pastry, white rice, white bread, crackers).

- To satisfy sugar cravings, eat dark chocolate, a handful of nuts, raw vegetables, desserts made with fruit or a couple of dates.

- Eat more fruit purée (dates, prunes), sweet-tasting vegetables (carrots, sweet potatoes), nuts and seeds.

- Don't add sugar to your coffee or tea. Just get used to it without sugar.

- Read labels and avoid foods that include sugar and its synonyms (glucose, fructose, sucrose) in the first three ingredients.

FOODS TO CHOOSE

Fruit
Pineapple, blueberries, blackberries, black currants, strawberries, kiwi, mango, papaya, peaches, pears, apples.

Vegetables
Garlic, asparagus, broccoli, celery, cabbage (green, kale or Brussels sprouts), squash, pumpkin, carrots, spinach, onion, sweet potato, avocado.

Fatty fish and seafood
Herring, mackerel, sardines, salmon, anchovies, tuna, trout, crab, oysters, shrimp.

Legumes
Lentils of all sorts, chickpeas, red beans.

Grains
Buckwheat, millet, quinoa, brown rice.

Nuts and grains (unsalted)
Brazil nuts, almonds, sunflower seeds, ground flaxseeds, hemp seeds, chia seeds, pumpkin seeds.

Herbs and spices
Cilantro, turmeric, ginger, cinnamon, cumin, cayenne pepper.

Oils
Extra virgin olive oil, nut oil, coconut oil.

Enriched soy and almond milk

Probiotics
Yogurt, fermented dairy products (depending on your tolerance).

Green tea

Red wine (in moderation)
Italian Cabernet Sauvignon, American Pinot Noir, Swiss Merlot.

FOODS TO AVOID

Fat
Cheese with over 20% m.f., cream, butter, fatty meats, cold cuts.

Refined sugar
Refined enriched flour, pastry, white rice, white bread, crackers.

Oils
Soybean oil, corn oil, sunflower seed oil.

Offal
Liver, kidneys.

Fatty meats
Pork, goose, certain cuts of lamb and beef.

Processed products containing hydrogenated fats
Crackers, cookies, granola bars and other packaged baked goods.

FOOD RECOMMENDATIONS
for gout

- Avoid red wine, game and seafood, which are rich in purines.

- Limit your consumption of sugary drinks (such as soft drinks) and foods rich in fructose, to reduce the level of uric acid.

- Choose fruits and vegetables rich in vitamin C, nuts and whole grains.

- Eat three pieces of fruit and 2 cups (500 ml) of vegetables per day. Plan at least one vegetarian meal a week, and ideally, one vegetarian meal a day.

- Spread your protein, carbohydrates and fats over the day.

- Drink 8 to 12 cups (2 to 3 l) of liquids per day, half of them in the form of water, to help eliminate uric acid.

- Coffee is fine. Regular, moderate consumption likely has a slightly protective effect.

- Limit your consumption of alcohol to a single drink a day and no more than three a week. Alcohol (particularly beer, whiskey, gin, vodka and rum) is one of the main risk factors for the disease.

- Don't overdo it. A calorie intake that regularly exceeds the body's needs increases the level of uric acid in the blood.

- Watch your weight, because being overweight can aggravate attacks of gout. If you are obese, losing weight gradually and slowly is advised, because it can lower the level of uric acid.

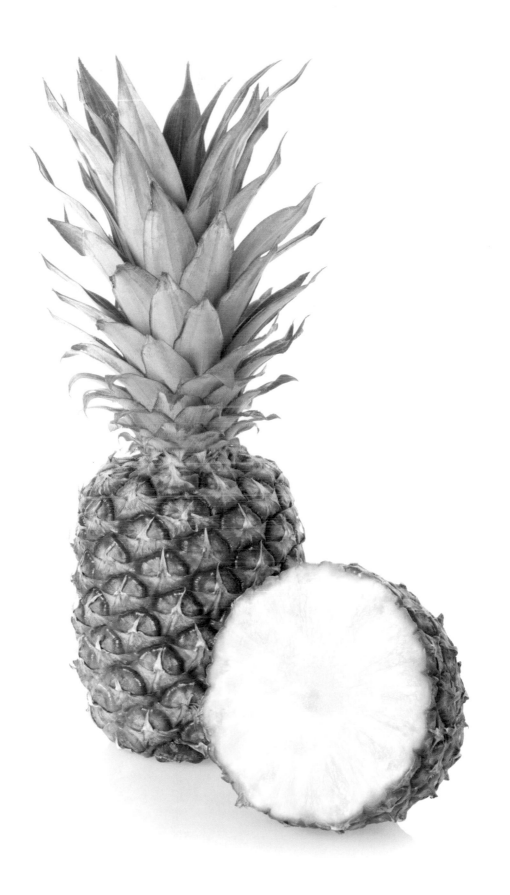

21 DAYS
OF MENUS

The following menus were designed using the latest data from the scientific literature.

Don't be afraid to vary quantities depending on how hungry you are. You can also combine menu items in different ways for endless variations.

Be your own chef and add a personal touch to the recipes to suit your tastes.

If you are vegetarian or vegan and don't eat animal or dairy products, we recommend taking a vitamin and mineral supplement and talking about it with your dietitian.

The emphasis in these menus is on nutrient density. Every recipe was designed for its nutritional value, so every one contains fruit or vegetables and food eaten raw and fresh. We encourage including as many plant-based foods in your diet as possible and limiting the consumption of red meat and processed food.

Have one of the following drinks as a snack after a meal or before going to bed: Anti-Inflammatory Water (see page 60), lemon water with mint, green tea with ginger, cinnamon coffee or green tea with star anise.

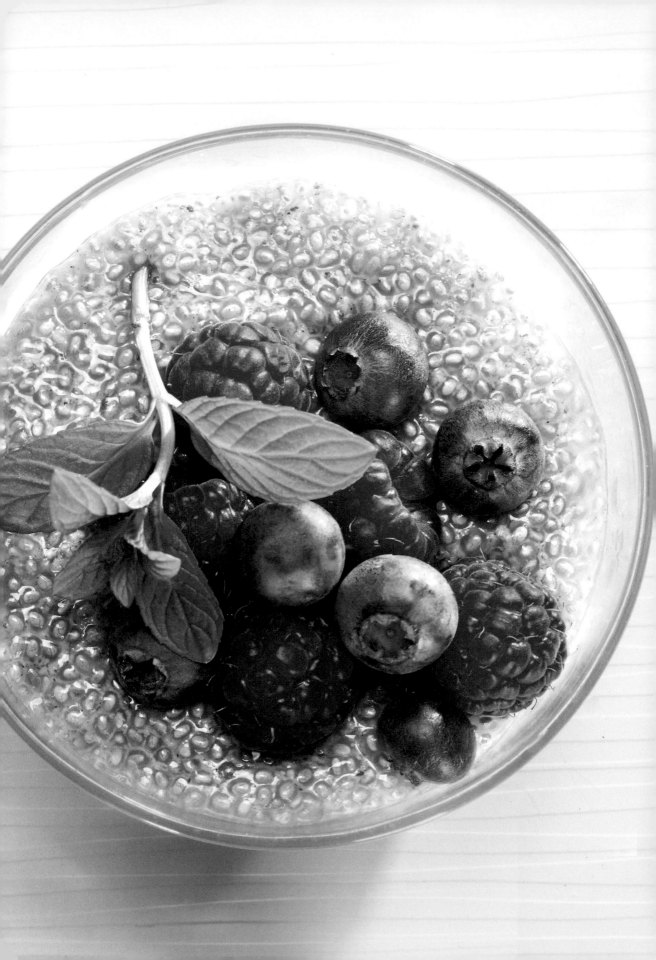

BREAKFAST

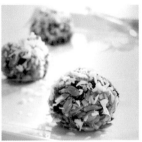

1 Flourless, Bakeless Anti-Inflammatory Ball (p. 68)
1 cup (250 ml) milk or plant-based milk
1 apple

Snack
Morning Snack (p. 70)
½ cup (125 ml) blueberries

LUNCH

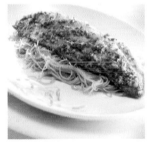

Rice Vermicelli with Pesto and Fish (p. 111)
Quick and Easy Kale Salad (p. 86)
1 kiwi or 2 clementines

Snack
Veggie Pâté, your choice (p. 76 and 79)
4 Buckwheat Flax Crackers (p. 80)

DINNER

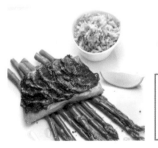

Gingery Sweet Potato Soup (p. 89)
Salmon Fillets with Anti-Inflammatory Spices (p. 112)
Versatile Salad (p. 90)

Snack
¼ cup (60 ml) Healthy Hummus (p. 82)
served with broccoli and carrots

DAY 2

BREAKFAST

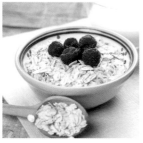

⅓ cup (80 ml) oat flakes with ½ cup (125 ml) milk or plant-based milk (almond or other)

A few walnuts
½ cup (125 ml) raspberries

Snack
1 celery stalk
1 tbsp almond butter

LUNCH

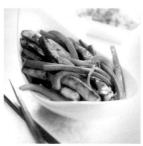

Asian Tofu and Turkey Stir-Fry (p. 114) served with ½ cup (125 ml) quinoa

Summer Fruit Salad with Chia Seeds (p. 144)

Snack
1 apple
A dozen almonds

DINNER

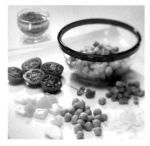

2 Indiana Salmon Cakes (p. 116) served with ½ cup (125 ml) cooked brown rice

Indian Salad (p. 92)

Snack
1 cup (250 ml) papaya
2 tbsp sunflower seeds

DAY 3

BREAKFAST

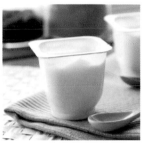

1 yogurt
2 tbsp sunflower seeds
⅓ cup (80 ml) kasha (roasted buckwheat seeds)
½ grapefruit

Snack
½ cup (125 ml) berries
1 tbsp chia seeds

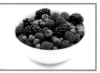

LUNCH

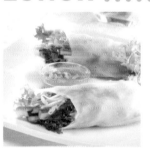

2 Spring Rolls (p. 118)
Kale Chips (p. 84)
1 kiwi

Snack
1 slice whole-grain bread
1 tbsp almond butter

DINNER

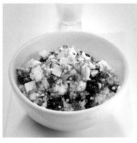

Gingery Sweet Potato Soup (p. 89)
5 Vegetarian Makis (p. 121)
Quinoa Salad with Cucumber, Avocado
and Pistachios (p. 94)

Snack
¼ cup (60 ml) mixed unsalted nuts

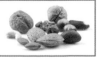

DAY 4

BREAKFAST

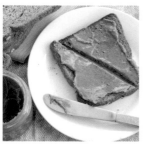

1 slice whole-grain bread
1 tbsp nut butter
1 small banana

Snack
1 Flourless, Bakeless
Anti-Inflammatory Ball (p. 68)

LUNCH

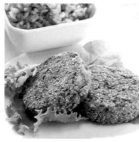

2 Indiana Salmon Cakes (p. 116)
served with ½ cup (125 ml) cooked brown rice

Fennel and Orange Salad (p. 96)
2 kiwis

Snack
Veggie Pâté, your choice (p. 76 and 79)
4 Buckwheat Flax Crackers (p. 80)

DINNER

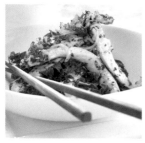

Turkey with Basil Pesto and Cabbage (p. 122)
Buckwheat Salad with Pomegranate
and Edamame (p. 98)

Snack
¼ cup (60 ml) silken tofu or plain yogurt
¼ cup (60 ml) mixed unsalted nuts
1 small banana

DAY 5

BREAKFAST

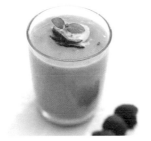

1 smoothie, your choice (p. 62, 64, 67)
¼ cup (60 ml) mixed unsalted nuts

Snack
Veggie Pâté, your choice (p. 76 and 79)
4 Buckwheat Flax Crackers (p. 80)

LUNCH

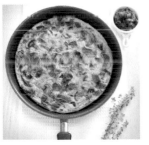

Fiesta Vegetable Frittata (p. 124)
served with ½ cup (125 ml) rice or quinoa
and ½ cup (125 ml) raw vegetables

20 cherries

Snack
1 yogurt
A dozen almonds
Summer Fruit Salad with Chia Seeds (p. 144)

DINNER

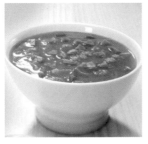

Gingery Carrot Soup (p. 101)
Chicken with Mango Salsa (p. 126)
Versatile Salad (p. 90)
1 pear

Snack
4 Buckwheat Flax Crackers (p. 80)
1 tbsp peanut butter
1 small banana

DAY 6

BREAKFAST

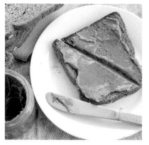

1 slice whole-grain bread
1 tbsp peanut butter
1 orange

Snack
1 Healthy Truffle (p. 69)

LUNCH

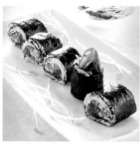

5 Vegan Makis (p. 121)
served with 1 cup (250 ml) green salad

1 Anti-Inflammatory Quinoa Drop (p. 146)
1 cup (250 ml) papaya

Snack
Veggie Pâté, your choice (p. 76 and 79)
1 slice whole-grain bread

DINNER

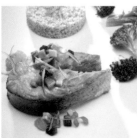

Salmon with Avocado and Citrus Salsa (p. 129)
served with broccoli
1 yogurt
Flourless, Bakeless Cinnamon Apple Crisp (p. 148)

Snack
1 Flourless, Bakeless
Anti-Inflammatory Ball (p. 68)

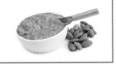

DAY 7

BREAKFAST ....

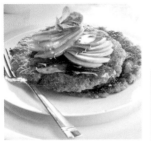

1 or 2 Pancakes with Pear and Cinnamon (p. 72)
A dozen almonds
½ cup (125 ml) raspberries

Snack
1 stalk celery
1 tbsp almond butter

LUNCH ....

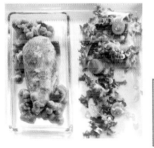

Easy Peasy Indian Chicken (p. 130)
served with 1 cup (250 ml) green salad

½ cup (125 ml) pineapple

Snack
3 squares (1 oz/30 g) 85% dark chocolate
1 apple

DINNER ....

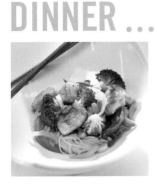

Rice Vermicelli with Salmon and Ginger (p. 132)
Fennel and Orange Salad (p. 96)
1 Surprising Melt-In-Your-Mouth Brownie (p. 151)

Snack
1 yogurt
½ cup (125 ml) blueberries

DAY 8

BREAKFAST

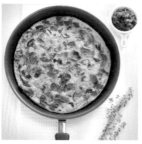

Fiesta Vegetable Frittata (p. 124)
1 slice whole-grain bread
1 orange

> **Snack**
> 1 yogurt
> 1 apple sprinkled with cinnamon

LUNCH

Salmon with Avocado and Citrus Salsa (p. 129)
served with ½ cup (125 ml) quinoa

Versatile Salad (p. 90)

Summer Fruit Salad with Chia Seeds (p. 144)

> **Snack**
> 1 banana
> A dozen almonds

DINNER

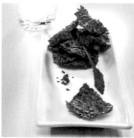

2 Spring Rolls (p. 118)
served with ½ cup (125 ml) cooked brown rice

Kale Chips (p. 84)
15 grapes

> **Snack**
> 1 yogurt
> ¼ cup (60 ml) pumpkin seeds

DAY 9

BREAKFAST

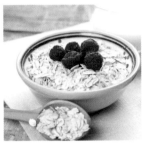

⅓ cup (80 ml) oat flakes with ½ cup (125 ml) milk or plant-based milk (almond or other)

A few walnuts

½ cup (125 ml) berries

> **Snack**
> Veggie Pâté, your choice (p. 76 and 79)
> 4 Buckwheat Flax Crackers (p. 80)

LUNCH

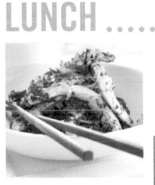

Gingery Carrot Soup (p. 100)

Turkey with Basil Pesto and Cabbage (p. 122) served with 1 cup (250 ml) green salad

1 pear

> **Snack**
> 1 Healthy Truffle (p. 69)

DINNER

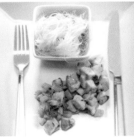

Chicken with Mango Salsa (p. 126) served with ⅓ cup (80 ml) brown rice vermicelli

Indian Salad (p. 92)

> **Snack**
> 1 slice whole-grain bread
> 1 tbsp nut butter
> 1 small banana

DAY 10

BREAKFAST

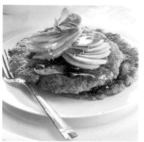

1 or 2 Pancakes with Pear and Cinnamon (p. 72)
A dozen almonds
1 small banana

Snack
Quick and Easy Smoothie (p. 67)

LUNCH

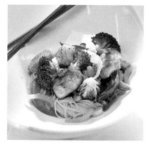

Rice Vermicelli with Salmon and Ginger (p. 132)
Fennel and Orange Salad (p. 96)
1 apple

Snack
¼ cup (60 ml) Healthy Hummus (p. 82)
served with broccoli and cauliflower

DINNER

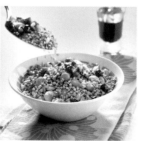

Italian Salad with Chickpeas and Quinoa (p. 102)
Flourless, Bakeless Cinnamon Apple Crisp (p. 148)

Snack
1 yogurt
½ cup (125 ml) blueberries

DAY 11

BREAKFAST

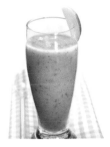

1 smoothie, your choice (p. 62, 64, 67)
A few walnuts

Snack
1 yogurt
½ cup (125 ml) pineapple

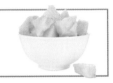

LUNCH

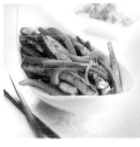

Gingery Sweet Potato Soup (p. 89)

Asian Tofu and Turkey Stir-Fry (p. 114)
served with ⅓ cup (80 ml) brown rice vermicelli

1 cup (250 ml) papaya

Snack
1 smoothie, your choice (p. 62, 64, 67)

DINNER

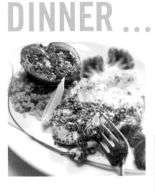

Fish Fillets with Fines Herbes (p. 134)
served with ½ cup (125 ml) cooked brown rice

Quick and Easy Kale Salad (p. 86)
1 orange

Snack
1 Flourless, Bakeless
Anti-Inflammatory Ball (p. 68)

DAY 12

BREAKFAST

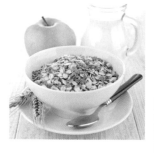

⅓ cup (80 ml) oat flakes with ½ cup (125 ml) milk or plant-based milk (almond or other)

A few walnuts

1 apple

Snack
Veggie Pâté, your choice (p. 76 and 79)
4 Buckwheat Flax Crackers (p. 80)

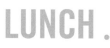

LUNCH

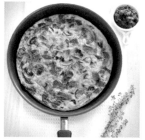

Fiesta Vegetable Frittata (p. 124)
Quick and Easy Kale Salad (p. 86)
1 orange

Snack
1 Flourless, Bakeless
Anti-Inflammatory Ball (p. 68)

DINNER

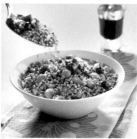

Buckwheat Salad with Pomegranate
and Edamame (p. 98)

1 small banana

Snack
1 Anti-Inflammatory Quinoa Drop (p. 146)

DAY 13

BREAKFAST

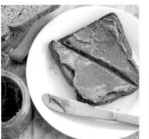

2 slices whole-grain bread
1 tbsp almond butter
1 banana

Snack
1 yogurt
2 clementines

LUNCH

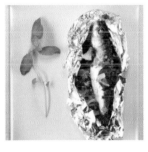

Fish en Papillote (p. 136)
Pineapple Quinoa Salad with Turmeric Vinaigrette (p. 104)
Kale Chips (p. 84)
Summer Fruit Salad with Chia Seeds (p. 144)

Snack
¼ cup (60 ml) Healthy Hummus (p. 82)
served with broccoli and cauliflower

DINNER

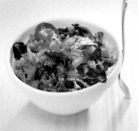

Gingery Carrot Soup (p. 101)
Rice Vermicelli with Salmon and Ginger (p. 132)
Versatile Salad (p. 90)

Snack
Veggie Pâté, your choice (p. 76 and 79)
4 Buckwheat Flax Crackers (p. 80)

DAY 14

BREAKFAST

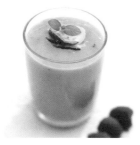

1 smoothie, your choice (p. 62, 64, 67)
¼ cup (60 ml) mixed unsalted nuts

Snack
1 Surprising Melt-In-Your-Mouth
Brownie (p. 151)

LUNCH

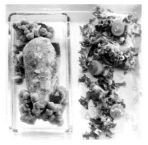

Easy Peasy Indian Chicken (p. 130)
Kale Chips (p. 84)
3 squares (1 oz/30 g) 85% dark chocolate

Snack
1 yogurt
A dozen almonds

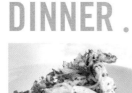

DINNER

Turkey with Basil Pesto and Cabbage (p. 122)
served with 1 cup (250 ml) green salad

1 slice whole-grain bread
2 clementines

Snack
Berry Easy Pudding (p. 74)
4 Buckwheat Flax Crackers (p. 80)

DAY 15

BREAKFAST

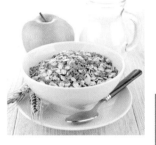

⅓ cup (80 ml) oat flakes with ½ cup (125 ml) milk or plant-based milk (almond or other)

A few walnuts

1 apple

> **Snack**
> 1 yogurt
> ¾ cup (180 ml) raspberries

LUNCH

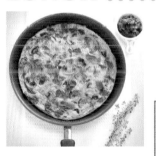

Fiesta Vegetable Frittata (p. 124)
1 slice whole-grain bread
Quick and Easy Kale Salad (p. 86)
½ cup (125 ml) blueberries

> **Snack**
> ¼ cup (60 ml) Healthy Hummus (p. 82)
> served with raw vegetables

DINNER

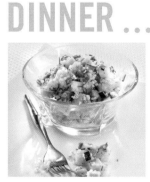

Summer Quinoa (p. 106)
Flourless, Bakeless Cinnamon Apple Crisp (p. 148)

> **Snack**
> 1 Anti-Inflammatory Quinoa Drop (p. 146)

DAY 16

BREAKFAST

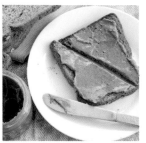

1 slice whole-grain bread
1 tbsp nut butter
1 small banana

Snack
Veggie Pâté, your choice (p. 76 and 79)
4 Buckwheat Flax Crackers (p. 80)
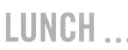

LUNCH

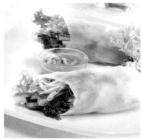

2 Spring Rolls (p. 118)
served with ½ cup (125 ml) cooked brown rice

Fennel and Orange Salad (p. 96)
1 yogurt, your choice

Snack
1 Flourless, Bakeless
Anti-Inflammatory Ball (p. 68)
½ cup (125 ml) blueberries

DINNER

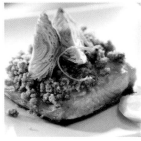

Gingery Carrot Soup (p. 101)
Nut-Crusted Salmon (p. 139)
Versatile Salad (p. 90)
1 orange

Snack
1 Healthy Truffle (p. 69)

DAY 17

BREAKFAST

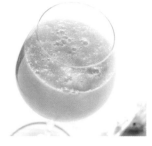

1 smoothie, your choice (p. 62, 64, 67)
¼ cup (60 ml) unsalted mixed nuts

> **Snack**
> 1 Surprising Melt-In-Your-Mouth
> Brownie (p. 151)

LUNCH

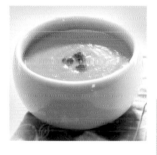

Gingery Sweet Potato Soup (p. 89)
5 Vegan Makis (p. 121)
served with 1 cup (250 ml) green salad

1 apple

> **Snack**
> Veggic Pâtć, your choicc (p. 76 and 79)
> 4 Buckwheat Flax Crackers (p. 80)

DINNER

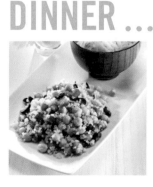

Italian Salad with Chickpeas and Quinoa (p. 102)
served with ½ cup (125 ml) kohlrabi

1 pear

> **Snack**
> ¼ cup (60 ml) Healthy Hummus (p. 82)
> served with celery and broccoli

DAY 18

BREAKFAST

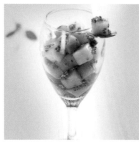

Summer Fruit Salad with Chia Seeds (p. 144)
1 Flourless, Bakeless Anti-Inflammatory Ball (p. 68)

> **Snack**
> Morning Snack (p. 70)

LUNCH

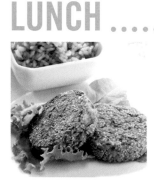

Indiana Salmon Cakes (p. 116)
Versatile Salad (p. 90)
1 slice whole-grain bread
3 squares (1 oz/30 g) 85% dark chocolate

> **Snack**
> 1 Healthy Truffle (p. 69)

DINNER

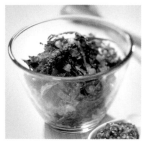

Quick and Easy Kale Salad (p. 86)
1 slice whole-grain bread

> **Snack**
> 1 Anti-Inflammatory Quinoa Drop (p. 146)

DAY 19

BREAKFAST

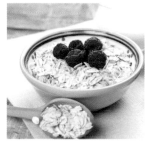

⅓ cup (80 ml) oat flakes with ½ cup (125 ml) milk or plant-based milk (almond or other)

A few walnuts
½ cup (125 ml) strawberries or raspberries

Snack
1 Healthy Truffle (p. 69)

LUNCH

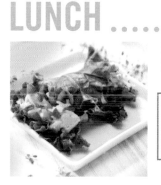

Kale Stuffed with Poultry and Basmati Rice (p. 141)
2 kiwis

Snack
1 slice whole-grain bread
1 tbsp almond butter

DINNER

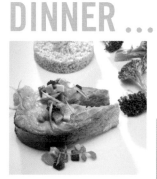

Salmon with Avocado and Citrus Salsa (p. 129)
served with Brussels sprouts

Flourless, Bakeless Cinnamon Apple Crisp (p. 148)

Snack
1 yogurt
½ cup (125 ml) blueberries

DAY 20

BREAKFAST

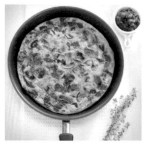

Fiesta Vegetable Frittata (p. 124)
½ grapefruit

Snack
1 slice whole-grain bread
1 tbsp peanut butter

LUNCH

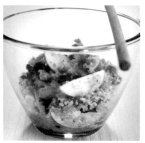

Quinoa Apple Salad (p. 108)
1 yogurt
2 tbsp sunflower seeds

Snack
¼ cup (60 ml) Healthy Hummus (p. 82)
served with raw vegetables

DINNER

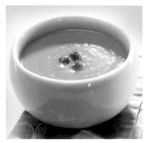

Gingery Sweet Potato Soup (p. 89)
Fennel and Orange Salad (p. 96)
3 squares (1 oz/30 g) 85% dark chocolate

Snack
1 Flourless, Bakeless
Anti-Inflammatory Ball (p. 68)

1 apple

DAY 21

BREAKFAST

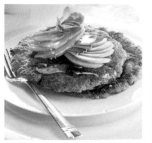

1 or 2 Pancakes with Pear and Cinnamon (p. 72)
A few walnuts
½ cup (125 ml) blueberries

Snack
¼ cup (60 ml) Healthy Hummus (p. 82)
served with broccoli and cauliflower

LUNCH

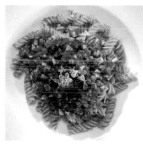

Meatless Bolognese Sauce (p. 143)
served with ½ cup (125 ml) whole wheat pasta
and 1 cup (250 ml) green salad

1 cup (250 ml) milk or plant-based milk (almond or other)
2 kiwis

Snack
Veggie Pâté, your choice (p. 76 and 79)
4 Buckwheat Flax Crackers (p. 80)

DINNER

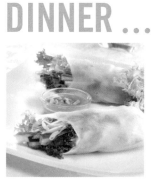

4 Spring Rolls (p. 118)
served with 1 cup (250 ml) green salad

Flourless, Bakeless Cinnamon Apple Crisp (p. 148)

Snack
Berry Easy Pudding (p. 74)

RECIPES
47 HEALTHY IDEAS

The following recipes contain ARTHRITIS INFO boxes with information about the anti-inflammatory benefits of certain foods. This will help you identify the best foods for your health.

DRINKS

Anti-Inflammatory Water 60
Incredible Green Smoothies.............62
Anti-Inflammatory Smoothie 64
Quick and Easy Smoothies 67

BREAKFASTS AND SWEET SNACKS

Flourless, Bakeless
Anti-Inflammatory Balls....................68
Healthy Truffles..............................69
Morning Snack 70
Pancakes with Pear
   and Cinnamon............................72
Berry Easy Pudding 74

APPETIZERS, SIDES AND SAVORY SNACKS

Delectable Veggie Pâté........................76
Root Vegetable Pâté...........................79
Buckwheat Flax Crackers....................80
Healthy Hummus 82
Kale Chips 84

SOUPS AND SALADS

Quick and Easy Kale Salad 86
Gingery Sweet Potato Soup 89
Versatile Salad..................................90
Indian Salad 92
Quinoa Salad with Cucumber,
   Avocado and Pistachios.................94
Fennel and Orange Salad 96
Buckwheat Salad with Pomegranate
   and Edamame............................98
Gingery Carrot Soup 101
Italian Salad with Chickpeas
   and Quinoa..................................102

Quinoa Pineapple Salad with
   Turmeric Vinaigrette 104
Summer Quinoa 106
Quinoa Apple Salad 108

MAIN COURSES

Rice Vermicelli with Pesto and Fish ...111
Salmon Fillets with
   Anti-Inflammatory Spices.............112
Asian Tofu and Turkey Stir-Fry........114
Indiana Salmon Cakes 116
Spring Rolls.................................118
Vegan Makis.................................121
Turkey with Basil Pesto
   and Cabbage.............................122
Fiesta Vegetable Frittata 124
Chicken with Mango Salsa..............126
Salmon with Avocado
   and Citrus Salsa.........................129
Easy Peasy Indian Chicken 130
Rice Vermicelli with Salmon
   and Ginger.................................132
Fish Fillets with Fines Herbes 134
Fish en Papillote 136
Nut-Crusted Salmon 139
Kale Stuffed with Poultry
   and Basmati Rice........................141
Meatless Bolognese Sauce.............143

DESSERTS

Summer Fruit Salad
   with Chia Seeds 144
Anti-Inflammatory Quinoa Drops......146
Flourless, Bakeless Cinnamon
   Apple Crisp................................148
Surprising Melt-In-Your-Mouth
   Brownies 151

ANTI-INFLAMMATORY
Water

MAKES: 4 cups (1 l) • PREPARATION: 2 minutes

INGREDIENTS

4 cups (1 l) water

Juice of 1 lemon

1 tsp minced fresh ginger

¼ tsp cayenne pepper

METHOD

In a bowl, combine water, lemon juice, ginger and cayenne pepper.

Mix well.

Serve chilled.

• • • • • • • • • • • • • •

TIP

This water will keep for 2 days in the fridge without losing its anti-inflammatory properties. You can drink as much of it as you like.

Nutrition Facts Per 1 cup (250 ml)	
Amount	% Daily Value
Calories 1	
Fat 0.1 g	0%
Saturated 0 g	0%
+ Trans 0 g	
Polyunsaturated 0 g	
Omega-6 0 g	
Omega-3 0 g	
Monounsaturated 0 g	
Cholesterol 0 mg	0%
Sodium 5 mg	0%
Potassium 10 mg	0%
Carbohydrate 0 g	0%
Fiber 0 g	0%
Sugars 0 g	
Protein 0.1 g	
Vitamin A 5 RE	0%
Vitamin C 0 mg	0%
Calcium 6 mg	0%
Iron 0.1 mg	0%
Phosphorous 1 mg	0%

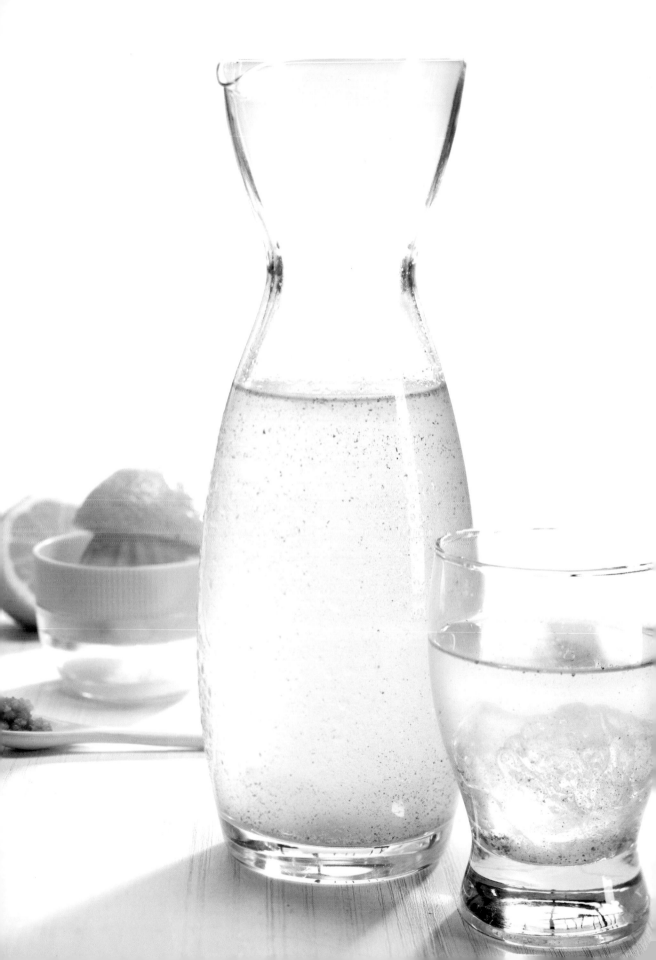

INCREDIBLE GREEN
Smoothies

2 servings • PREPARATION: 5 minutes

INGREDIENTS

1 cup (250 ml) pineapple cubes

1 small pear, peeled and cored

1 small ripe banana
or 2 chopped dates

½ cup (125 ml) spinach or 1 kale leaf

1 tbsp almond or other nut butter

2 cups (500 ml) green tea or water

METHOD

In a blender, place fruit, spinach and almond butter. Add tea. Blend to a smooth purée.

Add water to achieve desired consistency.

• • • • • • • • • • • • • •

VARIATION

Instead of pineapple, you can use 1 cup (250 ml) papaya or 1 cup (250 ml) fresh or frozen mango.

ARTHRITIS INFO

Bromelin, an enzyme found in pineapple, appears to inhibit the production of prostaglandins, which are the source of inflammation. Eating fresh pineapple regularly (1 to 2 cups/250 to 500 ml a day) can relieve painful joints.

Nutrition Facts Per serving	
Amount	% Daily Value
Calories 210	
Fat 5 g	8%
Saturated 0.5 g	3%
+ Trans 0 g	
Polyunsaturated 1 g	
Omega-6 1 g	
Omega-3 0.1 g	
Monounsaturated 3 g	
Cholesterol 0 mg	0%
Sodium 15 mg	1%
Potassium 500 mg	14%
Carbohydrate 38 g	13%
Fiber 5 g	20%
Sugars 23 g	
Protein 3 g	
Vitamin A 83 RE	8%
Vitamin C 40 mg	70%
Calcium 55 mg	6%
Iron 1 mg	8%
Phosphorous 73 mg	6%

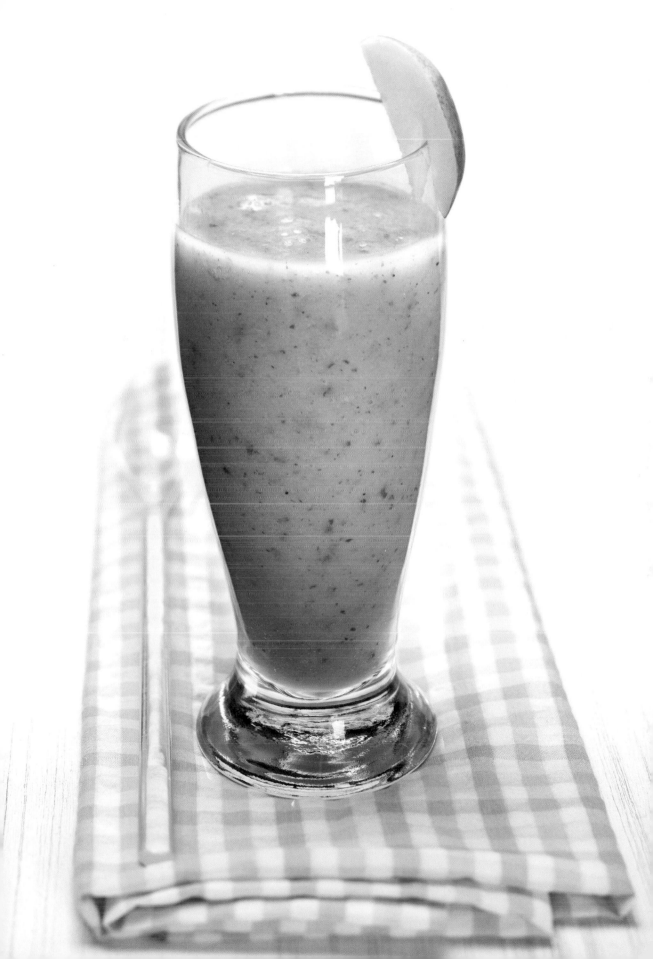

ANTI-INFLAMMATORY
Smoothie

1 serving • PREPARATION: 5 minutes

INGREDIENTS

½ pineapple, cut in large dice

2 celery stalks, cut in pieces

1 tsp grated fresh ginger

1 cup (250 ml) water (approx.)

METHOD

In a blender, place pineapple cubes, celery pieces and ginger. Add water and purée.

Add more water to achieve desired consistency and serve chilled.

Nutrition Facts
Per serving

Amount	% Daily Value
Calories 70	
Fat 0.3 g	0%
Saturated 0 g	0%
+ Trans 0 g	
Polyunsaturated 0.1 g	
Omega-6 0.1 g	
Omega-3 0 g	
Monounsaturated 0 g	
Cholesterol 0 mg	0%
Sodium 55 mg	2%
Potassium 310 mg	9%
Carbohydrate 17 g	6%
Fiber 3 g	12%
Sugars 12 g	
Protein 1 g	
Vitamin A 35 RE	4%
Vitamin C 45 mg	70%
Calcium 44 mg	4%
Iron 0.5 mg	4%
Phosphorous 26 mg	2%

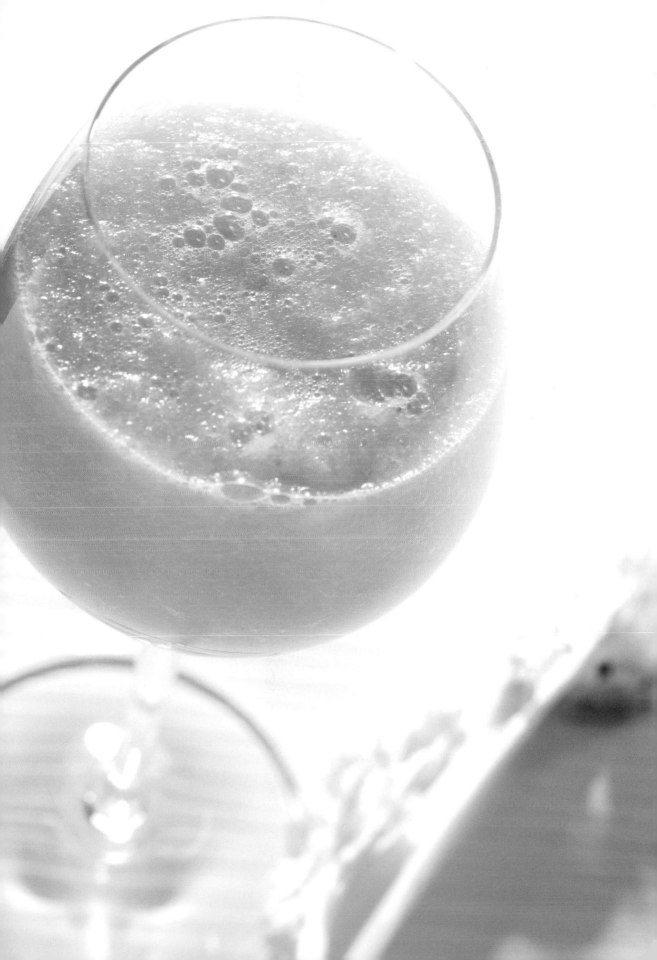

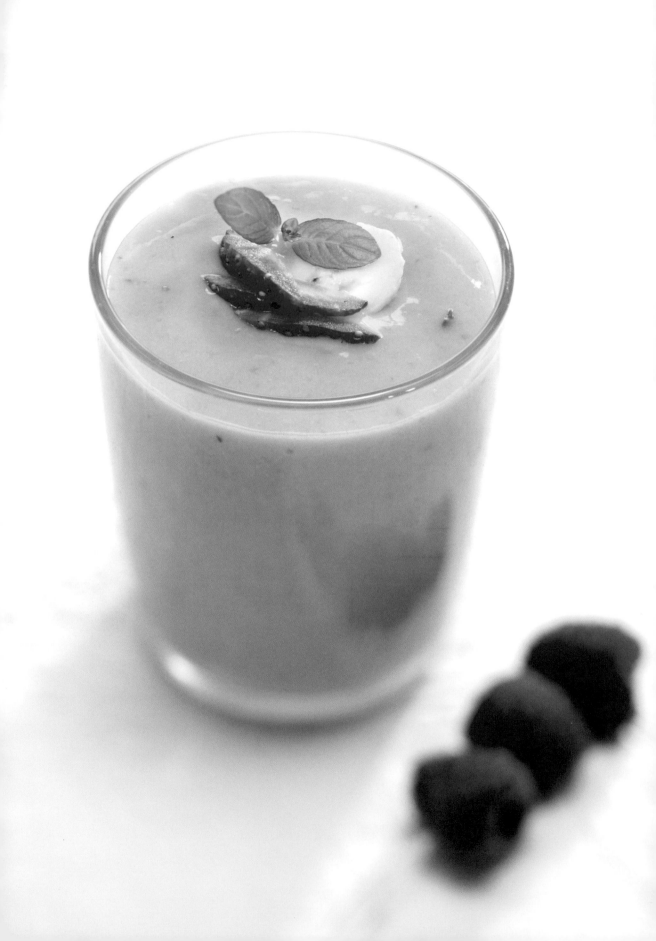

3 servings • PREPARATION: 5 minutes

METHOD

In a blender, place banana and frozen berries. Add liquid. Blend for 2 minutes.

Serve chilled.

INGREDIENTS

1 very ripe banana

2 cups (500 ml) frozen berries

1 cup (250 ml) almond milk, soy milk or milk

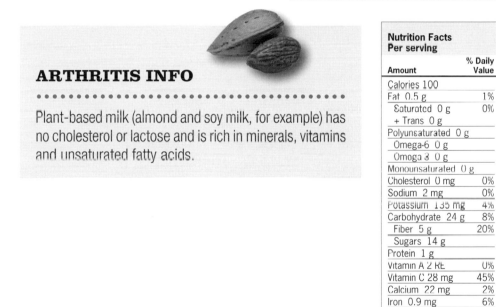

ARTHRITIS INFO

• •

Plant-based milk (almond and soy milk, for example) has no cholesterol or lactose and is rich in minerals, vitamins and unsaturated fatty acids.

**Nutrition Facts
Per serving**

Amount	% Daily Value
Calories 100	
Fat 0.5 g	1%
Saturated 0 g	0%
+ Trans 0 g	
Polyunsaturated 0 g	
Omega-6 0 g	
Omega-3 0 g	
Monounsaturated 0 g	
Cholesterol 0 mg	0%
Sodium 2 mg	0%
Potassium 135 mg	4%
Carbohydrate 24 g	8%
Fiber 5 g	20%
Sugars 14 g	
Protein 1 g	
Vitamin A 2 RE	0%
Vitamin C 28 mg	45%
Calcium 22 mg	2%
Iron 0.9 mg	6%
Phosphorous 8 mg	0%

FLOURLESS, BAKELESS
Anti-Inflammatory Balls

12 balls • PREPARATION: 10 minutes • REFRIGERATION TIME: 2 hours

INGREDIENTS

1 cup (250 ml) unsalted sunflower seeds, shelled

1 cup (250 ml) raisins, finely chopped

1 cup (250 ml) dates, finely chopped

Zest of 1 lemon

⅓ cup (80 ml) grated unsweetened coconut + 2 tbsp for coating

1 tsp ground cinnamon

2 tbsp honey or maple syrup

METHOD

In a large bowl, combine seeds, raisins, dates, lemon zest, ⅓ cup (80 ml) coconut, cinnamon and honey or maple syrup.

Shape into 12 balls, pressing firmly. Sprinkle with remaining coconut.

Refrigerate for 2 hours.

Nutrition Facts Per ball	
Amount	% Daily Value
Calories 190	
Fat 8 g	12%
Saturated 1.5 g	8%
+ Trans 0 g	
Polyunsaturated 4.5 g	
Omega-6 4.5 g	
Omega-3 0 g	
Monounsaturated 1.5 g	
Cholesterol 0 mg	0%
Sodium 3 mg	0%
Potassium 280 mg	8%
Carbohydrate 27 g	9%
Fiber 4 g	16%
Sugars 20 g	
Protein 3 g	
Vitamin A 1 RE	0%
Vitamin C 1 mg	2%
Calcium 25 mg	2%
Iron 1.4 mg	10%
Phosphorous 165 mg	15%

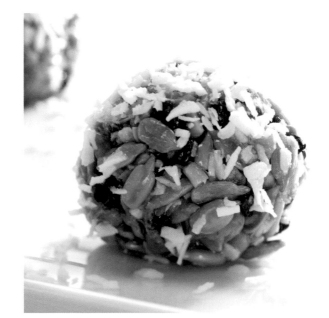

12 truffles • PREPARATION: 20 minutes

METHOD

In a food processor, combine dates, pecans, walnuts, cocoa, cinnamon and water.

With food processor running, add maple syrup in a thin stream. Mix to form a smooth paste.

Use your hands to shape paste into a dozen balls and roll in grated coconut.

Refrigerate as needed before serving.

INGREDIENTS

10 dates, chopped

½ cup (125 ml) pecans, coarsely chopped

½ cup (125 ml) walnuts, coarsely chopped

¼ cup (60 ml) cocoa powder

1 tsp ground cinnamon

1 tbsp water

2 tbsp maple syrup

½ cup (125 ml) grated unsweetened coconut

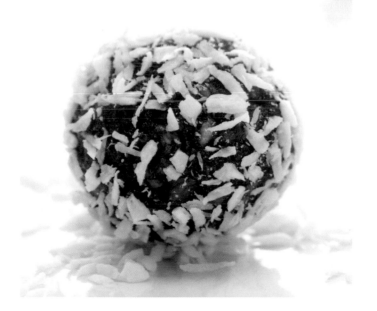

Nutrition Facts Per truffle		
Amount		% Daily Value
Calories 110		
Fat 7 g		11%
Saturated 2 g		10%
+ Trans 0 g		
Polyunsaturated 3 g		
Omega-6 2.5 g		
Omega-3 0.4 g		
Monounsaturated 2.5 g		
Cholesterol 0 mg		0%
Sodium 20 mg		1%
Potassium 130 mg		4%
Carbohydrate 10 g		3%
Fiber 2 g		8%
Sugars 7 g		
Protein 2 g		
Vitamin A 1 RE		0%
Vitamin C 0 mg		0%
Calcium 17 mg		2%
Iron 0.8 mg		6%
Phosphorous 47 mg		4%

MORNING

Snack

2 servings • PREPARATION: 15 minutes

INGREDIENTS

¼ cup (60 ml) whole chia seeds

1 tbsp almond or peanut butter

4 dates, chopped, or 1 small ripe banana

Pinch ground cinnamon

1 cup (250 ml) water

½ cup (125 ml) your choice berries (blueberries, raspberries, etc.)

¼ cup (60 ml) pistachios or sunflower seeds

1 tsp maple syrup (optional)

METHOD

In a bowl, combine chia seeds, almond or peanut butter, dates or banana, cinnamon and water.

Let stand at least 10 minutes to thicken.

To serve, garnish with berries, pistachios or sunflower seeds, and maple syrup, if desired.

• • • • • • • • • • • • • •

TIP

Prepare your morning snack the night before.

Nutrition Facts Per serving	
Amount	**% Daily Value**
Calories 400	
Fat 21 g	32%
Saturated 2.5 g	13%
+ Trans 0 g	
Polyunsaturated 10 g	
Omega-6 5 g	
Omega-3 5 g	
Monounsaturated 7 g	
Cholesterol 0 mg	0%
Sodium 10 mg	0%
Potassium 390 mg	11%
Carbohydrate 42 g	14%
Fiber 14 g	56%
Sugars 14 g	
Protein 10 g	
Vitamin A 18 RE	2%
Vitamin C 21 mg	35%
Calcium 241 mg	20%
Iron 4.8 mg	35%
Phosphorous 416 mg	40%

ARTHRITIS INFO

• •

Blueberries contain anthocyanins, which are rich in antioxidant and anti-inflammatory properties.

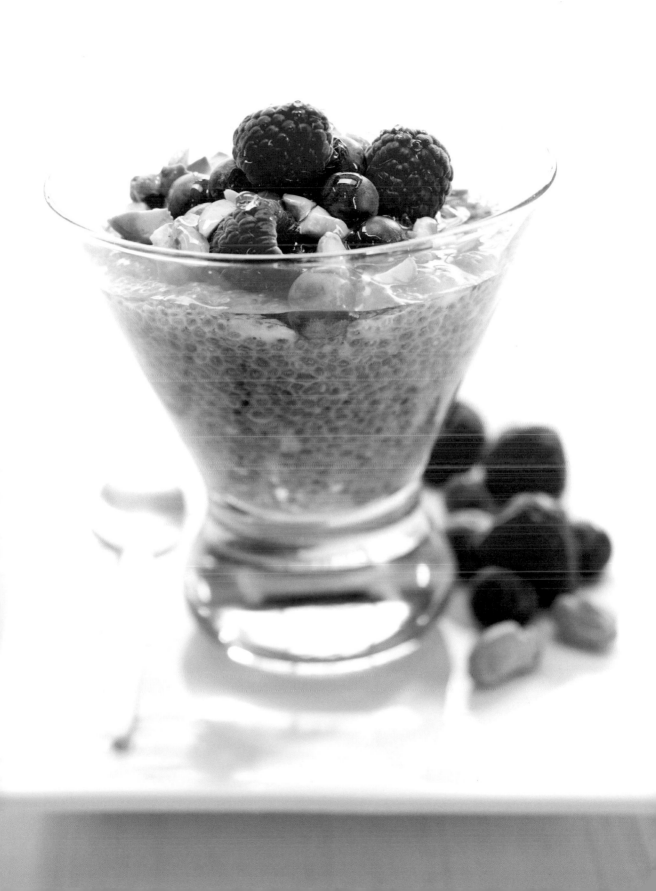

PANCAKES WITH PEAR
and Cinnamon

2 pancakes • PREPARATION: 15 minutes • COOKING TIME: 15 minutes

INGREDIENTS

½ cup (125 ml) quinoa flakes

¼ cup (60 ml) whole chia seeds

1 pear, peeled, cored and cut in pieces, divided

Pinch ground ginger

Pinch ground nutmeg

1 cup (250 ml) water

½ tsp ground cinnamon

1 tsp maple syrup or honey (optional)

METHOD

In a bowl, combine quinoa flakes, chia seeds, half the pear (reserve the other half for garnish), ginger, nutmeg and water. Let stand for 10 minutes to thicken.

In a lightly greased skillet, cook pancakes over medium heat about 3 minutes per side or until light golden.

Garnish with pieces of reserved pear and sprinkle with cinnamon. Drizzle with maple syrup or honey, if desired.

Nutrition Facts Per pancake	
Amount	% Daily Value
Calories 350	
Fat 10 g	15%
Saturated 0.5 g	3%
+ Trans 0 g	
Polyunsaturated 5 g	
Omega-6 1.5 g	
Omega-3 4 g	
Monounsaturated 0.5 g	
Cholesterol 0 mg	0%
Sodium 15 mg	1%
Potassium 150 mg	4%
Carbohydrate 55 g	18%
Fiber 14 g	56%
Sugars 12 g	
Protein 9 g	
Vitamin A 6 RE	0%
Vitamin C 4 mg	6%
Calcium 164 mg	15%
Iron 4.5 mg	30%
Phosphorous 218 mg	20%

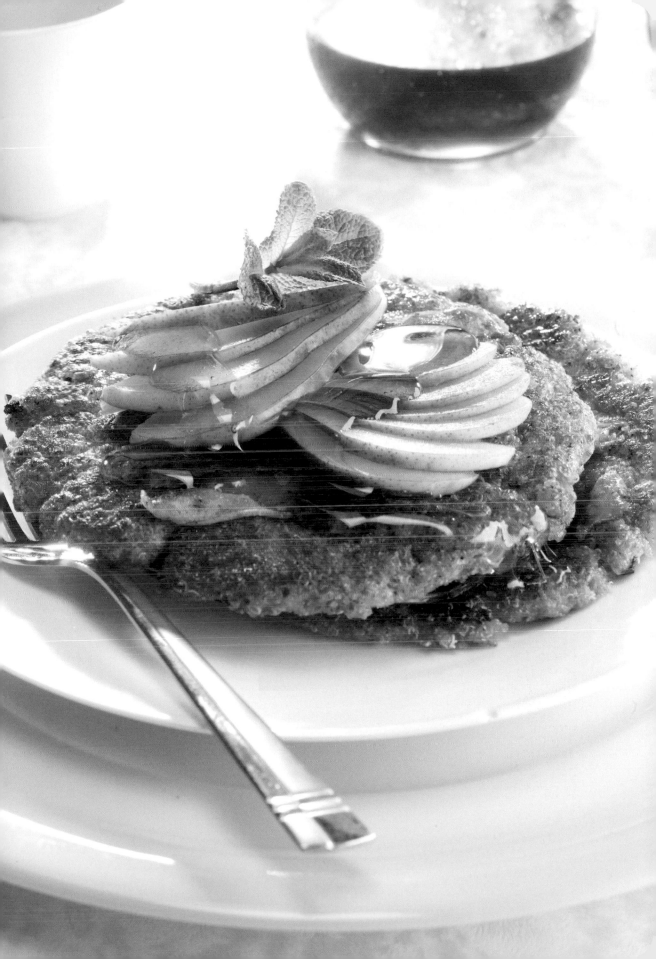

BERRY EASY
Pudding

4 servings • PREPARATION: 15 minutes • REFRIGERATION TIME: 2 hours

INGREDIENTS

2 tbsp almond butter

½ cup (125 ml) whole white chia seeds

1 tsp honey or maple syrup

2 cups (500 ml) water

Cinnamon to taste

2 cups (500 ml) berries for garnish

METHOD

In a bowl, whisk together almond butter, seeds, honey or maple syrup, water and cinnamon.

Divide mixture into four dessert cups. Let stand 5 minutes. Refrigerate 2 hours (overnight is best), stirring two or three times so seeds absorb liquid.

Garnish with berries before serving.

• • • • • • • • • • • • • •

TIP

For a thicker pudding, increase the amount of chia seeds in the recipe.

Nutrition Facts Per serving	
Amount	% Daily Value
Calories 290	
Fat 15 g	23%
Saturated 1.5 g	8%
+ Trans 0 g	
Polyunsaturated 8 g	
Omega-6 3 g	
Omega-3 6 g	
Monounsaturated 3.5 g	
Cholesterol 0 mg	0%
Sodium 10 mg	0%
Potassium 120 mg	3%
Carbohydrate 32 g	11%
Fiber 12 g	48%
Sugars 2 g	
Protein 7 g	
Vitamin A 16 RE	2%
Vitamin C 35 mg	60%
Calcium 225 mg	20%
Iron 4.6 mg	35%
Phosphorous 338 mg	30%

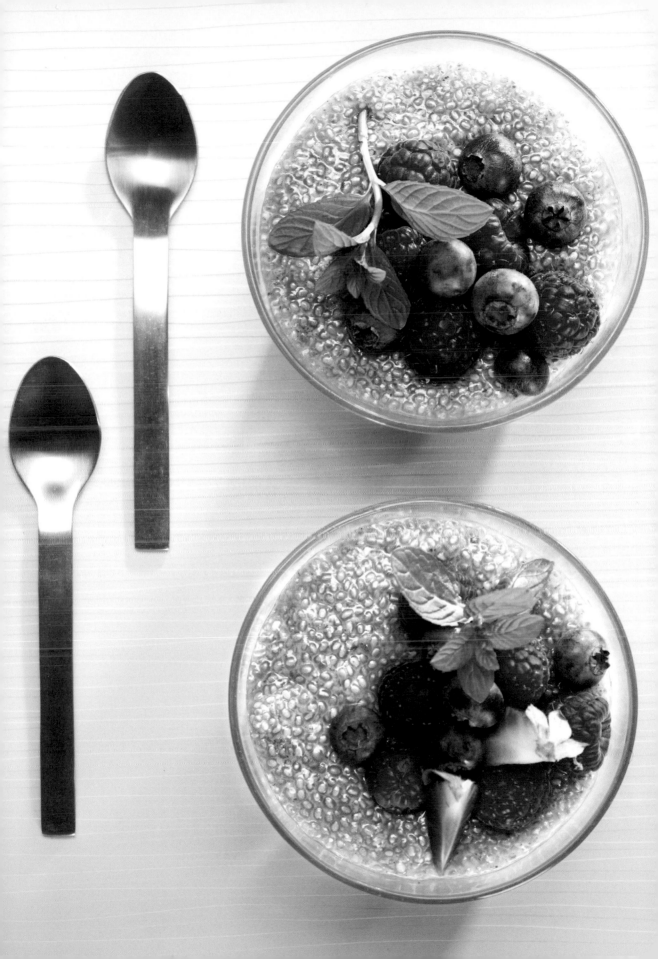

DELECTABLE VEGGIE
Pâté

12 servings • PREPARATION: 10 minutes • COOKING TIME: 1 hour

INGREDIENTS

1 cup (250 ml) cooked lentils or other legume

1 cup (250 ml) ground sunflower seeds

½ cup (125 ml) ground chia seeds

1 tbsp Brewer's yeast

1 large onion, finely sliced

2 garlic cloves, finely chopped

¼ cup (60 ml) olive or other oil

2 tbsp lemon juice

½ cup (125 ml) warm water

2 tsp miso, or salt to taste

½ tsp dried thyme

2 tsp ground cumin

½ tsp freshly ground pepper

½ tsp ground sage

METHOD

Preheat oven to 200°F (100°C).

Lightly grease an ovenproof dish with sides.

In a bowl, combine ingredients and transfer to prepared ovenproof dish. Bake for 1 hour with oven door open a crack.

Remove from oven and let stand for 10 minutes.

Serve with crackers, Buckwheat Flax Crackers (p. 80), whole-grain bread or celery.

• • • • • • • • • • • • • •

TIP

Store refrigerated for up to 1 week.

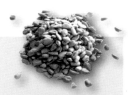

ARTHRITIS INFO

• •

Sunflower seeds contain plenty of vitamin E, vitamin B6 and copper. You only need a small handful daily to get all the benefits.

Nutrition Facts Per serving		
Amount		% Daily Value
Calories 220		
Fat 15 g		23%
Saturated 1.5 g		8%
+ Trans 0 g		
Polyunsaturated 7 g		
Omega-6 5 g		
Omega-3 2 g		
Monounsaturated 1.5 g		
Cholesterol 0 mg		0%
Sodium 40 mg		2%
Potassium 190 mg		5%
Carbohydrate 14 g		5%
Fiber 6 g		24%
Sugars 1 g		
Protein 6 g		
Vitamin A 2 RE		0%
Vitamin C 3 mg		4%
Calcium 94 mg		8%
Iron 3 mg		20%
Phosphorous 280 mg		25%

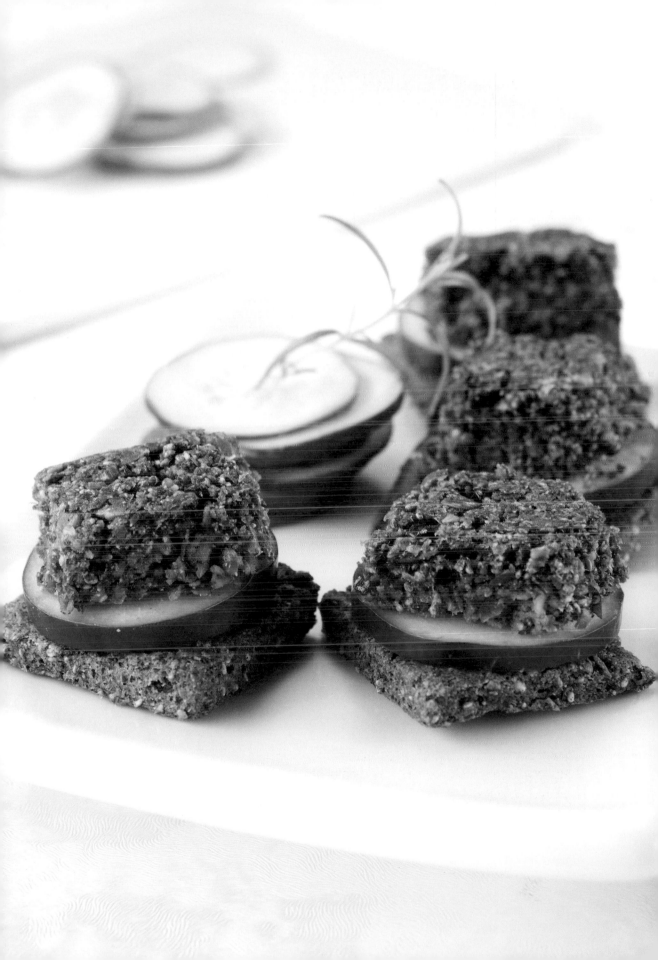

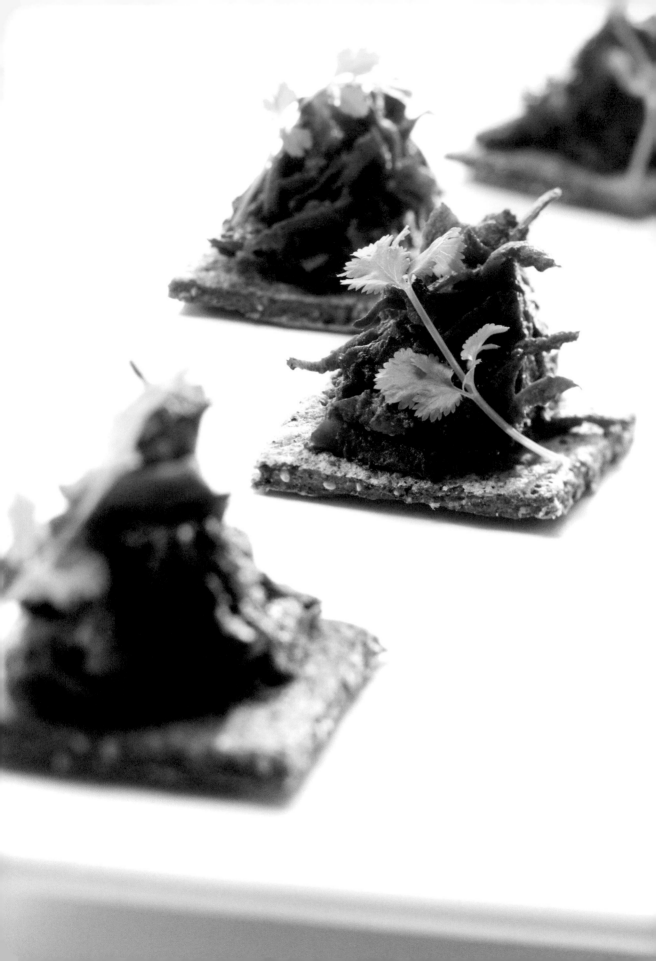

12 servings • PREPARATION: 10 minutes • COOKING TIME: 45 minutes

METHOD

Preheat oven to 320°F (160°C).

In a food processor, grind sunflower seeds.

In a bowl, combine sunflower seeds with remaining ingredients. Pour mixture into a 10-inch (25 cm) square Pyrex dish and bake on middle rack of preheated oven, 40 to 45 minutes.

Let pâté cool for 10 minutes before cutting.

Serve with crackers, Buckwheat Flax Crackers (p. 80), whole-grain bread or celery.

. . . .

TIP

Store refrigerated for up to 1 week.

INGREDIENTS

1½ cups (375 ml) sunflower seeds

¼ cup (60 ml) sesame seeds

½ cup (125 ml) buckwheat flour

1 onion, finely chopped

2 cloves garlic, finely chopped

1 large beet, grated

1 large carrot, grated

1 turnip, grated

1 tsp ground cumin

2 tsp ground coriander

1 cup (250 ml) warm water

¼ cup (60 ml) tamari

Nutrition Facts Per serving	
Amount	% Daily Value
Calories 180	
Fat 12 g	18%
Saturated 1.5 g	8%
+ Trans 0 g	
Polyunsaturated 7 g	
Omega-6 7 g	
Omega-3 0 g	
Monounsaturated 2.5 g	
Cholesterol 0 mg	0%
Sodium 370 mg	15%
Potassium 240 mg	7%
Carbohydrate 13 g	4%
Fiber 4 g	16%
Sugars 2 g	
Protein 5 g	
Vitamin A 82 RE	8%
Vitamin C 2 mg	4%
Calcium 35 mg	4%
Iron 2.1 mg	15%
Phosphorous 270 mg	25%

BUCKWHEAT FLAX
Crackers

12 small or 24 mini crackers (approx.) • PREPARATION: 15 minutes • COOKING TIME: 20 minutes

INGREDIENTS

½ cup (125 ml) buckwheat flour

2 tsp whole chia seeds

2 tsp ground flaxseeds

1 tsp curry powder

½ tsp baking powder

¾ cup (180 ml) almond milk

2 tsp extra virgin olive oil

METHOD

Preheat oven to 200°F (100°C).

In a bowl, blend flour, chia seeds, flaxseeds, curry powder, baking powder and almond milk to a smooth paste.

In a skillet, heat oil over medium heat and cook paste, 2 minutes per side. Transfer to a baking sheet and dry in preheated oven for 15 minutes.

Cut into 12 small or 24 mini crackers.

Serve crackers with veggie pâté or other topping, such as peanut or almond butter.

• • • • • • • • • • • • • •

TIP

Keep your chia seeds and flaxseeds in an airtight container in the fridge.

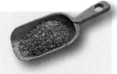

ARTHRITIS INFO

Chia seeds and flaxseeds are a good source of omega-3s, zinc, selenium and copper. Zinc and selenium are a dynamic duo of minerals for fighting arthritis.

Nutrition Facts Per 1 small cracker		% Daily
Amount		Value
Calories 15		
Fat 0.5 g		1%
Saturated 0.1 g		1%
+ Trans 0 g		
Polyunsaturated 0.2 g		
Omega-6 0.1 g		
Omega-3 0.2 g		
Monounsaturated 0.4 g		
Cholesterol 0 mg		0%
Sodium 10 mg		0%
Potassium 20 mg		1%
Carbohydrate 2 g		1%
Fiber 0 g		0%
Sugars 0 g		
Protein 0.4 g		
Vitamin A 1 RE		0%
Vitamin C 0 mg		0%
Calcium 10 mg		0%
Iron 0.2 mg		2%
Phosphorous 16 mg		2%

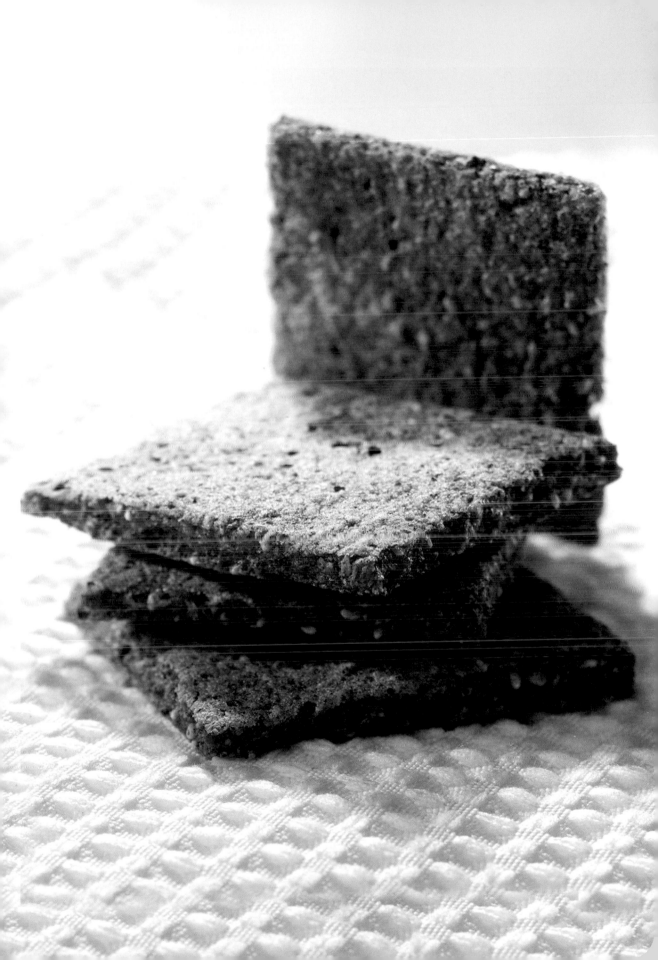

HEALTHY
Hummus

MAKES: 2 cups (500 ml) • PREPARATION: 10 minutes • COOKING TIME: 1 hour

INGREDIENTS

1 can (14 oz/398 ml) chickpeas, drained and rinsed

2 green onions, sliced

2 cloves garlic, chopped

2 tbsp lemon juice

6 tbsp olive oil

½ cup (125 ml) chopped parsley or cilantro (or a combination of both)

½ tsp ground cumin

¼ cup (60 ml) tahini (sesame paste)

1 tsp miso

METHOD

In a blender, combine all ingredients and purée.

If mixture is too thick, add water or lemon juice.

Refrigerate for 1 hour before serving.

Serve with raw vegetables (broccoli, carrots, cauliflower, celery, etc.) or Buckwheat Flax Crackers (p. 80).

Nutrition Facts Per ¼ cup (60 ml)		
Amount		**% Daily Value**
Calories 190		
Fat 13 g		20%
Saturated 2 g		10%
+ Trans 0 g		
Polyunsaturated 1.5 g		
Omega-6 1.5 g		
Omega-3 0 g		
Monounsaturated 1 g		
Cholesterol 0 mg		0%
Sodium 35 mg		1%
Potassium 170 mg		5%
Carbohydrate 13 g		4%
Fiber 3 g		12%
Sugars 2 g		
Protein 4 g		
Vitamin A 35 RE		4%
Vitamin C 9 mg		15%
Calcium 41 mg		4%
Iron 1.8 mg		15%
Phosphorous 104 mg		10%

ARTHRITIS INFO

Legumes (particularly chickpeas) have anti-inflammatory properties and are rich in fiber. They are good meat substitutes. In terms of protein, 1 cup (250 ml) of cooked legumes equals 3 oz (85 g) of meat.

KALE
Chips

4 servings • PREPARATION: 5 minutes • COOKING TIME: 8 minutes

INGREDIENTS

8 cups (2 l) kale

2 tsp olive oil

2 tsp tamari or soy sauce

METHOD

Preheat oven to 320°F (160°C) and lightly grease a baking sheet.

Cut kale leaves into the shape of chips. In a bowl, combine olive oil and tamari. Add kale and toss to coat.

Place kale pieces on prepared baking sheet and bake, about 8 minutes. Check regularly and remove from oven once crisp.

Serve kale chips as a side or a snack.

• • • • • • • • • • • • • •

VARIATION

Bake kale stems along with leaves. They're delicious.

Nutrition Facts Per serving	
Amount	% Daily Value
Calories 100	
Fat 3 g	5%
Saturated 0.4 g	2%
+ Trans 0 g	
Polyunsaturated 0.5 g	
Omega-6 0.2 g	
Omega-3 0.3 g	
Monounsaturated 0.1 g	
Cholesterol 0 mg	0%
Sodium 230 mg	10%
Potassium 640 mg	18%
Carbohydrate 14 g	5%
Fiber 3 g	12%
Sugars 3 g	
Protein 5 g	
Vitamin A 2177 RE	220%
Vitamin C 85 mg	140%
Calcium 192 mg	15%
Iron 2.5 mg	20%
Phosphorous 83 mg	8%

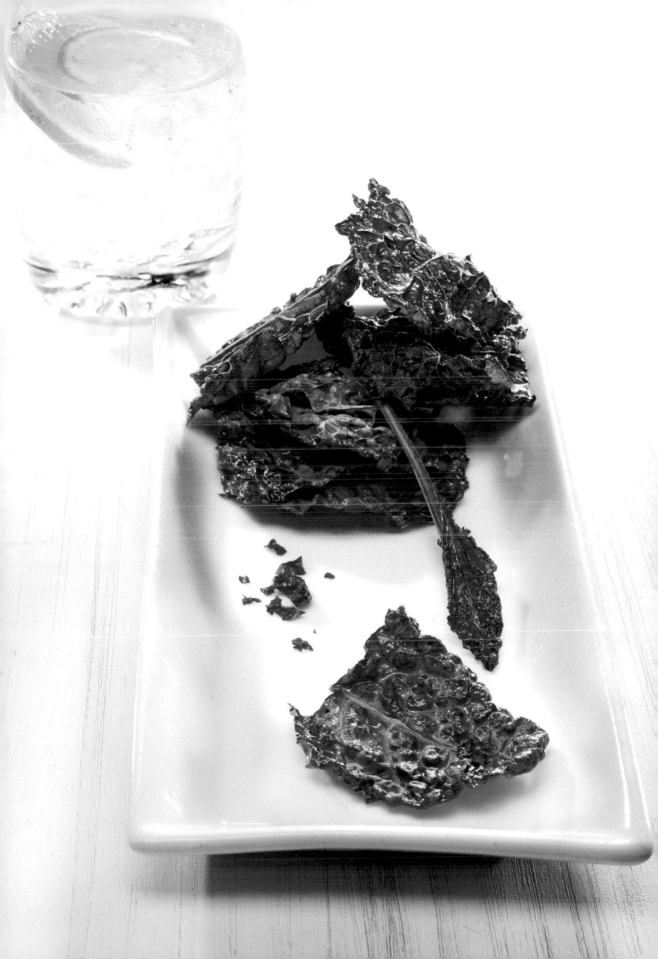

QUICK AND EASY KALE
Salad

2 servings • PREPARATION: 15 minutes

INGREDIENTS

2 cups (500 ml) kale, cut into thin strips

2 seedless clementines, peeled and diced

For the vinaigrette

1 tbsp lemon juice

1 tbsp rice vinegar

1 tbsp olive or sesame oil

1 tsp clementine zest

1 tsp miso

2 dates, chopped

1 tsp curry powder or turmeric

½ tsp grated fresh ginger

2 tsp toasted sesame seeds (optional)

METHOD

In a salad bowl, toss cabbage and clementines together.

In a small bowl, combine ingredients for vinaigrette.

When ready to serve, pour vinaigrette over salad and toss.

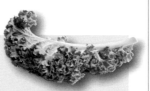

ARTHRITIS INFO

Kale is increasingly popular in nutritional therapy. It has a very high nutrient density and is rich in vitamins and other phytochemicals recommended for relieving symptoms of arthritis.

Nutrition Facts Per serving		
Amount		% Daily Value
Calories 100		
Fat 4.5 g		7%
Saturated 0.5 g		3%
+ Trans 0 g		
Polyunsaturated 0.5 g		
Omega-6 0.4 g		
Omega-3 0.1 g		
Monounsaturated 0.3 g		
Cholesterol 0 mg		0%
Sodium 70 mg		3%
Potassium 70 mg		3%
Carbohydrate 14 g		5%
Fiber 2 g		8%
Sugars 8 g		
Protein 2 g		
Vitamin A 574 RE		60%
Vitamin C 56 mg		90%
Calcium 71 mg		6%
Iron 1 mg		8%
Phosphorous 46 mg		4%

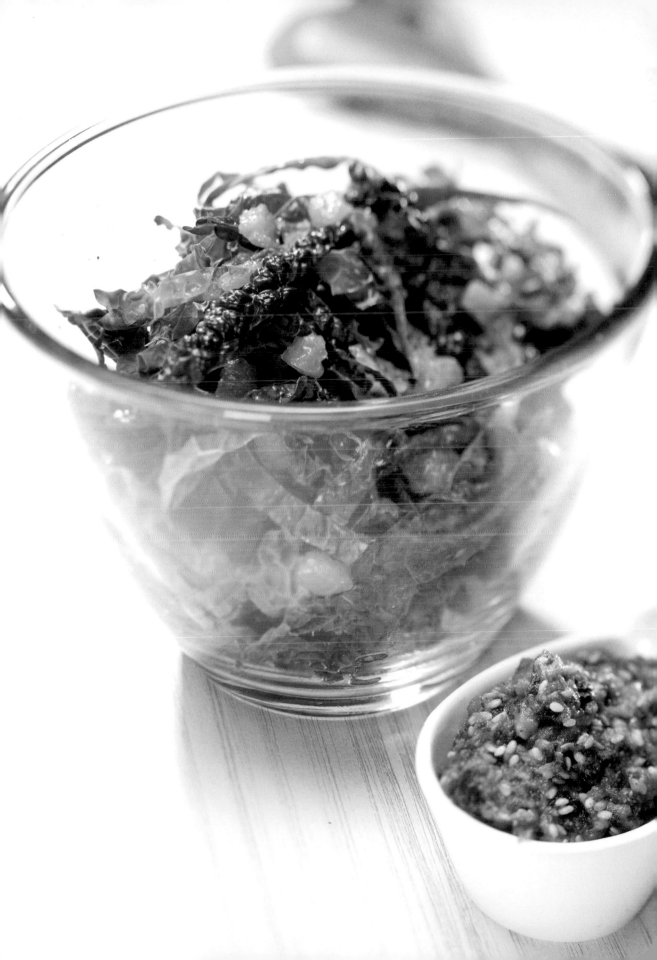

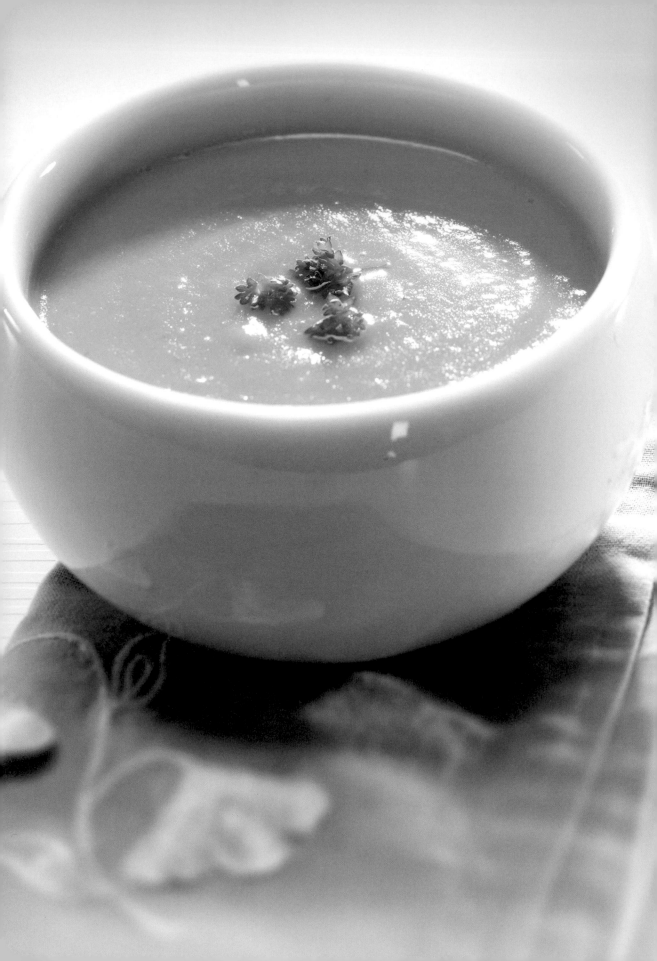

GINGERY SWEET POTATO
Soup

4 servings • PREPARATION: 5 minutes • COOKING TIME: 20 minutes

METHOD

In a skillet, heat oil over medium heat and sauté onion and garlic, stirring occasionally, for 2 minutes.

Add remaining ingredients, except miso and parsley, and bring to a boil.

Cover and simmer gently (reduce heat to low, if necessary) for 20 minutes or until sweet potatoes are tender.

Purée soup in a blender, if desired.

Add miso or salt, and garnish with parsley before serving.

INGREDIENTS

1 tsp olive or other oil

1 medium onion, finely chopped

1 clove garlic, sliced

4 cups (1 l) diced sweet potatoes

2 tsp grated fresh ginger

6 cups (1.5 l) vegetable broth

½ tsp dried thyme

½ tsp curry powder

Freshly ground pepper

2 tsp miso, or salt to taste

¼ cup (60 ml) chopped fresh parsley

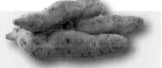

ARTHRITIS INFO

• •

Sweet potatoes are health allies because they are rich in beta-carotene, which is helpful in fighting the inflammation associated with rheumatoid arthritis.

Nutrition Facts Per serving		
Amount		% Daily Value
Calories 350		
Fat 2.5 g		4%
Saturated 0.5 g		3%
+ Trans 0 g		
Polyunsaturated 0.5 g		
Omega-6 0.5 g		
Omega-3 0 g		
Monounsaturated 0.1 g		
Cholesterol 0 mg		0%
Sodium 530 mg		22%
Potassium 1870 mg		53%
Carbohydrate 73 g		24%
Fiber 16 g		64%
Sugars 25 g		
Protein 8 g		
Vitamin A 4917 RE		490%
Vitamin C 30 mg		50%
Calcium 303 mg		30%
Iron 4.3 mg		30%
Phosphorous 240 mg		20%

VERSATILE
Salad

4 servings • PREPARATION: 15 minutes

INGREDIENTS

4 cups (1 l) mixed greens, arugula
or baby spinach

1 orange, finely diced

2 tbsp almonds or walnuts

For the vinaigrette

2 tbsp freshly squeezed orange juice

1 tbsp lemon juice

1 tbsp olive or other oil

2 tbsp chopped fresh basil,
dill or parsley

2 tsp mixed orange and lemon zest

1 tsp finely chopped fresh ginger

1 tsp miso, or salt to taste

METHOD

In a bowl, combine mixed greens, orange and almonds.

In a small bowl, combine ingredients for vinaigrette.

When ready to serve, pour vinaigrette over salad and toss.

Nutrition Facts Per serving	
Amount	% Daily Value
Calories 100	
Fat 5 g	8%
Saturated 0.5 g	3%
+ Trans 0 g	
Polyunsaturated 0.4 g	
Omega-6 0.4 g	
Omega-3 0 g	
Monounsaturated 1 g	
Cholesterol 0 mg	0%
Sodium 80 mg	3%
Potassium 140 mg	4%
Carbohydrate 10 g	3%
Fiber 3 g	12%
Sugars 6 g	
Protein 3 g	
Vitamin A 276 RE	30%
Vitamin C 48 mg	80%
Calcium 75 mg	6%
Iron 1.2 mg	8%
Phosphorous 26 mg	2%

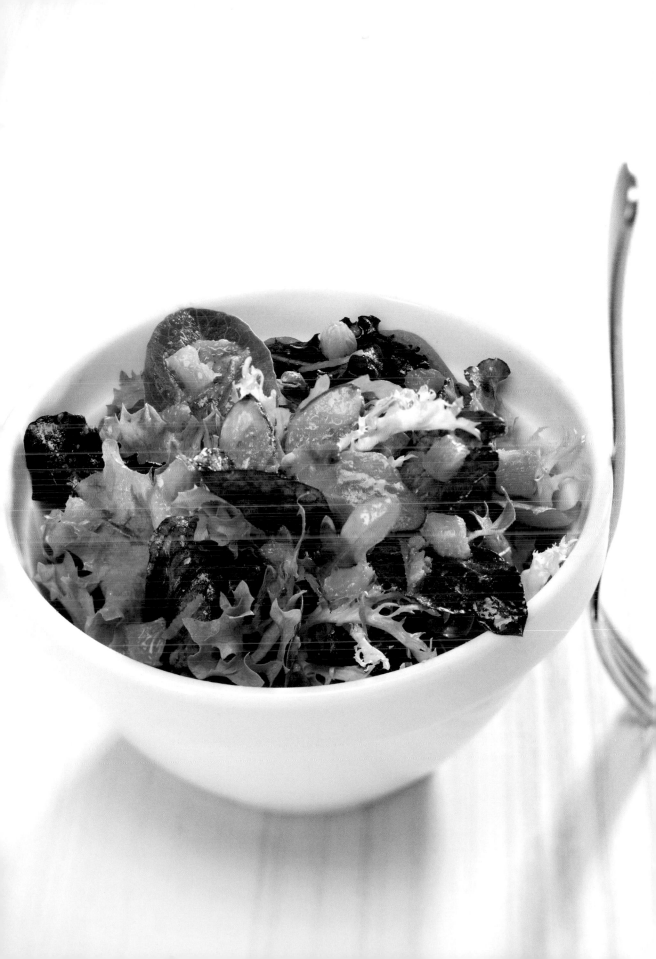

INDIAN
Salad

4 servings • PREPARATION: 15 minutes

INGREDIENTS

1 onion, chopped

2 cloves garlic, finely chopped

1 bell pepper, diced

1 carrot, peeled and finely diced

1 can (14 oz/398 ml) chickpeas, drained and rinsed

1 cup (250 ml) cherry tomatoes, halved

Freshly ground pepper and salt

For the vinaigrette

1 tbsp olive oil

Zest and juice of 1 lime

2 tsp honey

2 tsp cumin seeds

1 tsp curry powder

¼ cup (60 ml) roughly chopped fresh cilantro

METHOD

In a large bowl, combine salad ingredients.

In a small bowl, combine ingredients for vinaigrette.

Add vinaigrette to salad ingredients and toss well.

Let marinate for 10 minutes before serving.

Nutrition Facts Per serving		
Amount		**% Daily Value**
Calories 230		
Fat 6 g		9%
Saturated 0.5 g		3%
+ Trans 0 g		
Polyunsaturated 1 g		
Omega-6 1 g		
Omega-3 0.1 g		
Monounsaturated 0.5 g		
Cholesterol 0 mg		0%
Sodium 90 mg		4%
Potassium 610 mg		17%
Carbohydrate 36 g		12%
Fiber 6 g		24%
Sugars 11 g		
Protein 9 g		
Vitamin A 347 RE		35%
Vitamin C 59 mg		100%
Calcium 111 mg		10%
Iron 4.1 mg		30%
Phosphorous 182 mg		15%

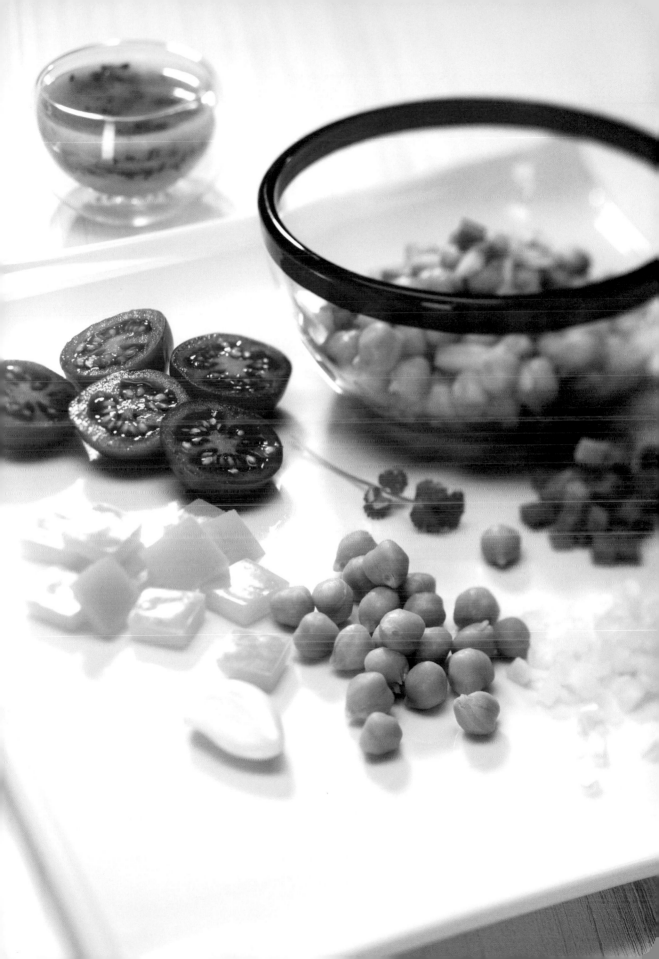

QUINOA SALAD WITH CUCUMBER,
Avocado and Pistachios

4 servings • PREPARATION: 10 minutes • COOKING TIME: 15 minutes

INGREDIENTS

1 cup (250 ml) uncooked quinoa, rinsed

2½ cups (625 ml) water

½ cucumber, diced

1 avocado, diced

¼ cup (60 ml) dried cranberries or cherries

½ cup (125 ml) pistachios

1 green onion, sliced

Fresh cilantro or parsley, to taste

For the vinaigrette

¼ cup (60 ml) olive oil

Juice of ½ orange

1 tbsp apple cider vinegar

Cayenne pepper

METHOD

In a medium saucepan, combine quinoa and water. Cover and bring to a boil. Reduce heat and simmer for 15 to 20 minutes or until liquid is absorbed. Let cool.

In a small bowl, whisk together ingredients for vinaigrette.

In a large bowl, combine cooled quinoa, cucumber, avocado, cranberries, pistachios, green onion and herbs. Toss with vinaigrette.

Nutrition Facts Per serving	
Amount	% Daily Value
Calories 410	
Fat 18 g	28%
Saturated 2 g	10%
+ Trans 0 g	
Polyunsaturated 4 g	
Omega-6 3.5 g	
Omega-3 0.1 g	
Monounsaturated 7 g	
Cholesterol 0 mg	0%
Sodium 25 mg	0%
Potassium 790 mg	22%
Carbohydrate 50 g	17%
Fiber 7 g	28%
Sugars 11 g	
Protein 11 g	
Vitamin A 25 RE	2%
Vitamin C 20 mg	35%
Calcium 87 mg	8%
Iron 6 mg	45%
Phosphorous 296 mg	25%

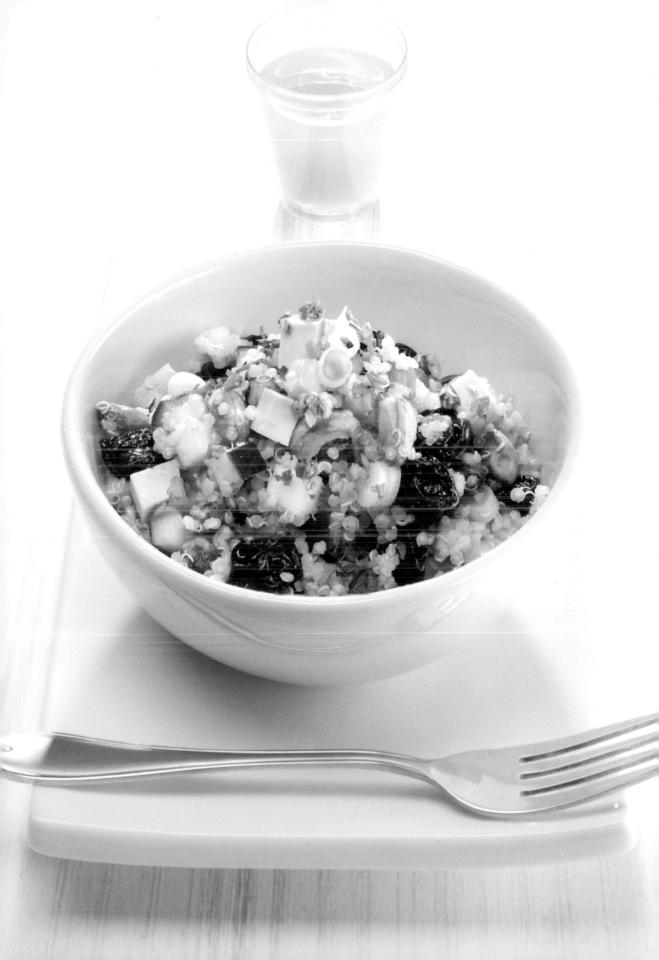

FENNEL AND ORANGE
Salad

4 servings • PREPARATION: 15 minutes

INGREDIENTS

2 cups (500 ml) fennel, cut into thin strips

1 seedless orange, peeled and diced

For the vinaigrette

2 tbsp lemon juice

1 tbsp olive or other oil

1 tsp orange zest

1 tsp miso

2 dates, chopped

1 tbsp chopped fresh cilantro

2 tbsp whole chia seeds

1 tsp honey or maple syrup (optional)

METHOD

In a bowl, combine fennel and orange.

In a small bowl, combine ingredients for vinaigrette.

When ready to serve, toss salad with vinaigrette.

Nutrition Facts Per serving	
Amount	**% Daily Value**
Calories 140	
Fat 6 g	9%
Saturated 0.5 g	3%
+ Trans 0 g	
Polyunsaturated 2 g	
Omega-6 0.5 g	
Omega-3 1.5 g	
Monounsaturated 0.2 g	
Cholesterol 0 mg	0%
Sodium 80 mg	3%
Potassium 350 mg	10%
Carbohydrate 18 g	6%
Fiber 6 g	24%
Sugars 8 g	
Protein 3 g	
Vitamin A 20 RE	2%
Vitamin C 38 mg	60%
Calcium 99 mg	8%
Iron 1.4 mg	10%
Phosphorous 108 mg	10%

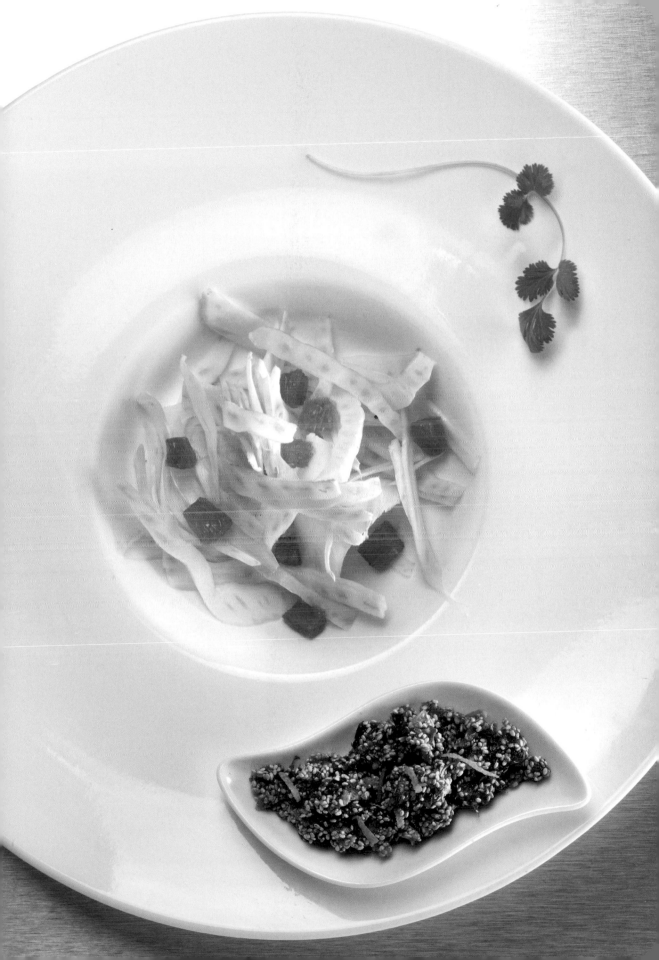

BUCKWHEAT SALAD
with Pomegranate and Edamame

4 servings • PREPARATION: 10 minutes

INGREDIENTS

1½ cups (375 ml) buckwheat, cooked

1 pomegranate, seeded

1 cup (250 ml) edamame (soybeans), cooked

¼ cup (60 ml) walnuts

¼ cup (60 ml) diced red onion

1 cup (250 ml) arugula

For the vinaigrette

2 tbsp extra virgin olive oil

1 tbsp balsamic vinegar

1 tbsp maple syrup

METHOD

In a large bowl, combine buckwheat, pomegranate, edamame, walnuts, red onion and arugula.

In a bowl, whisk together ingredients for vinaigrette.

Toss salad with vinaigrette and serve.

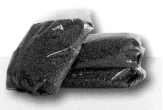

Nutrition Facts Per serving	
Amount	**% Daily Value**
Calories 490	
Fat 18 g	28%
Saturated 2.5 g	13%
+ Trans 0 g	
Polyunsaturated 4 g	
Omega-6 2.5 g	
Omega-3 0.5 g	
Monounsaturated 7 g	
Cholesterol 0 mg	0%
Sodium 10 mg	0%
Potassium 470 mg	14%
Carbohydrate 66 g	22%
Fiber 6 g	24%
Sugars 14 g	
Protein 17 g	
Vitamin A 57 RE	6%
Vitamin C 9 mg	15%
Calcium 74 mg	6%
Iron 3.7 mg	25%
Phosphorous 260 mg	25%

ARTHRITIS INFO

Buckwheat is a whole grain that is rich in fiber and contains no gluten. It is a good addition to an anti-inflammatory diet.

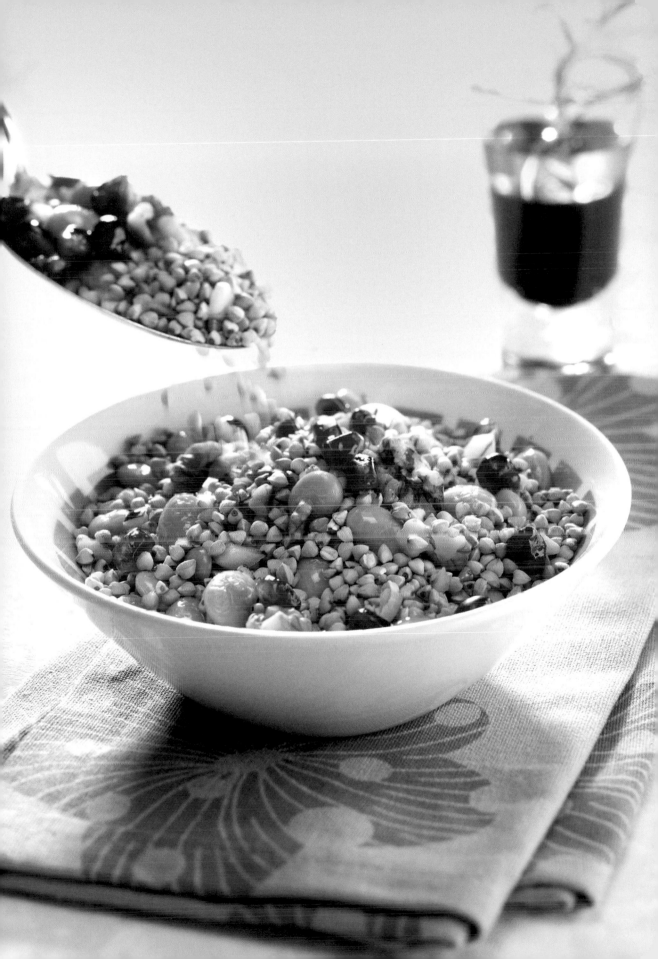

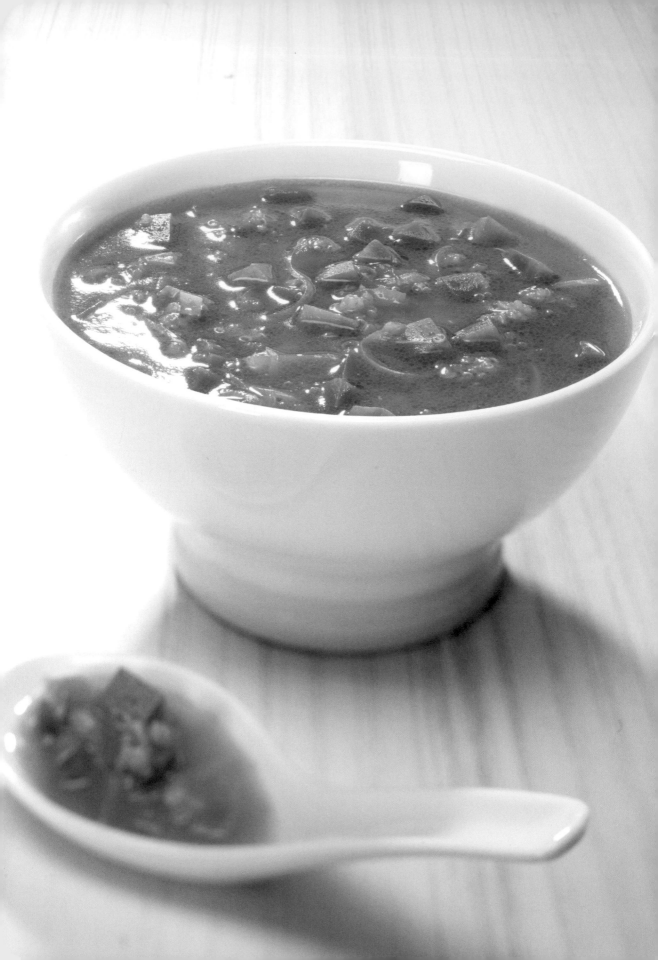

GINGERY CARROT
Soup

6 servings • PREPARATION: 15 minutes • COOKING TIME: 30 minutes

METHOD

In a large saucepan, heat oil over medium heat for a few seconds. Add onion, garlic, carrots and celery and sauté, stirring, about 4 minutes. Do not brown.

Add ginger, curry powder and orange zest. Cook, stirring, for 1 minute.

Add stock and quinoa. Cover, reduce heat to low and simmer, about 20 minutes.

Add orange juice and miso at the end of cooking. Stir and season.

Serve the soup alone or with kohlrabi.

• • • • • • • • • • • • • •

TIP

This soup pairs well with the mild vegetable kohlrabi.

INGREDIENTS

1 tbsp olive or other oil

1 onion, finely sliced

2 cloves garlic, finely chopped

3 cups (750 ml) diced peeled carrots

2 stalks celery, diced

2 tsp finely chopped fresh ginger

2 tsp curry powder

1 tsp orange zest

6 cups (1.5 l) vegetable stock

½ cup (125 ml) uncooked quinoa or rice

½ cup (125 ml) orange juice

1 tbsp miso, or salt to taste

Freshly ground pepper

Nutrition Facts Per serving	
Amount	**% Daily Value**
Calories 280	
Fat 4.5 g	7%
Saturated 0.5 g	3%
+ Trans 0 g	
Polyunsaturated 1 g	
Omega-6 1 g	
Omega-3 0 g	
Monounsaturated 0.3 g	
Cholesterol 0 mg	0%
Sodium 400 mg	17%
Potassium 1370 mg	39%
Carbohydrate 52 g	17%
Fiber 11 g	44%
Sugars 20 g	
Protein 7 g	
Vitamin A 2623 RE	260%
Vitamin C 29 mg	50%
Calcium 218 mg	20%
Iron 3.8 mg	25%
Phosphorous 217 mg	20%

ARTHRITIS INFO

• •

Carrots (like sweet potato) are health allies because they are rich in beta-carotene, which fights the inflammation associated with rheumatoid arthritis.

101

ITALIAN SALAD WITH CHICKPEAS
and Quinoa

4 servings • PREPARATION: 10 minutes • COOKING TIME: 20 minutes • REFRIGERATION TIME: 1 hour

INGREDIENTS

1 cup (250 ml) uncooked quinoa, rinsed

2½ cups (625 ml) water

2 cloves garlic, sliced

2 cups (500 ml) cooked chickpeas or other legume

⅓ cup (80 ml) diced fresh tomatoes

¼ cup (60 ml) black olives, roughly chopped

For the vinaigrette

¼ cup (60 ml) olive or other oil

2 tbsp lemon juice

2 tsp Dijon mustard

1 tsp chopped fresh tarragon or parsley

1 tsp miso

¼ tsp freshly ground pepper

1 tbsp honey

METHOD

In a medium saucepan, combine quinoa and water. Cover and bring to a boil. Reduce heat and simmer for 15 to 20 minutes or until liquid is absorbed. Let cool.

In a large bowl, combine ingredients for vinaigrette. Add garlic, chickpeas, tomatoes, olives and cooled quinoa. Combine.

Refrigerate for 1 hour before serving.

Serve salad alone or with kohlrabi.

• • • • • • • • • • • • •

TIP

This soup pairs well with the mild vegetable kohlrabi.

Nutrition Facts Per serving	
Amount	**% Daily Value**
Calories 390	
Fat 9 g	14%
Saturated 1 g	5%
+ Trans 0 g	
Polyunsaturated 2 g	
Omega-6 2 g	
Omega-3 0.1 g	
Monounsaturated 1.5 g	
Cholesterol 0 mg	0%
Sodium 210 mg	9%
Potassium 700 mg	20%
Carbohydrate 63 g	21%
Fiber 8 g	32%
Sugars 8 g	
Protein 15 g	
Vitamin A 10 RE	2%
Vitamin C 11 mg	20%
Calcium 112 mg	10%
Iron 7.4 mg	50%
Phosphorous 356 mg	30%

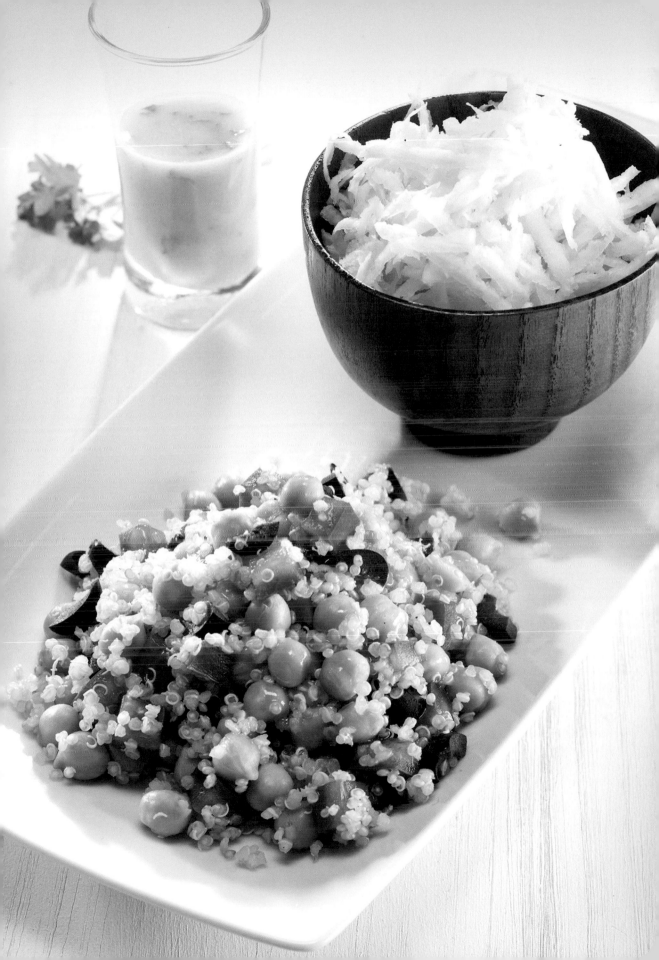

QUINOA PINEAPPLE SALAD
with Turmeric Vinaigrette

4 servings • PREPARATION: 15 minutes • COOKING TIME: 20 minutes

INGREDIENTS

1 cup (250 ml) uncooked quinoa, rinsed

2½ cups (625 ml) water

2½ cups (625 ml) diced pineapple

½ cup (125 ml) diced red onion

½ cup (125 ml) finely chopped cilantro or other herb

For the Tumeric Vinaigrette

3 tbsp olive oil

2 tbsp apple cider vinegar

2 tbsp maple syrup or honey

1 tsp turmeric

1 tsp curry powder

1 clove garlic, chopped

Freshly ground pepper

METHOD

In a medium saucepan, combine quinoa and water. Cover and bring to a boil. Reduce heat and simmer for 15 to 20 minutes or until liquid is absorbed. Let cool a little.

In a small bowl, vigorously whisk ingredients for vinaigrette together to emulsify.

In a large bowl, combine cooled quinoa with pineapple, onion and cilantro. Pour vinaigrette over salad and toss.

Serve chilled.

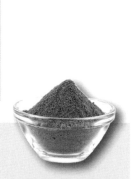

ARTHRITIS INFO

• •

Turmeric has proven anti-inflammatory properties. It is particularly effective at preventing inflammation.

Nutrition Facts Per serving	
Amount	% Daily Value
Calories 380	
Fat 13 g	20%
Saturated 1.5 g	8%
+ Trans 0 g	
Polyunsaturated 1 g	
Omega-6 1 g	
Omega-3 0.1 g	
Monounsaturated 1 g	
Cholesterol 0 mg	0%
Sodium 25 mg	1%
Potassium 720 mg	20%
Carbohydrate 57 g	19%
Fiber 6 g	24%
Sugars 18 g	
Protein 8 g	
Vitamin A 29 RE	2%
Vitamin C 62 mg	100%
Calcium 116 mg	10%
Iron 6.8 mg	50%
Phosphorous 228 mg	20%

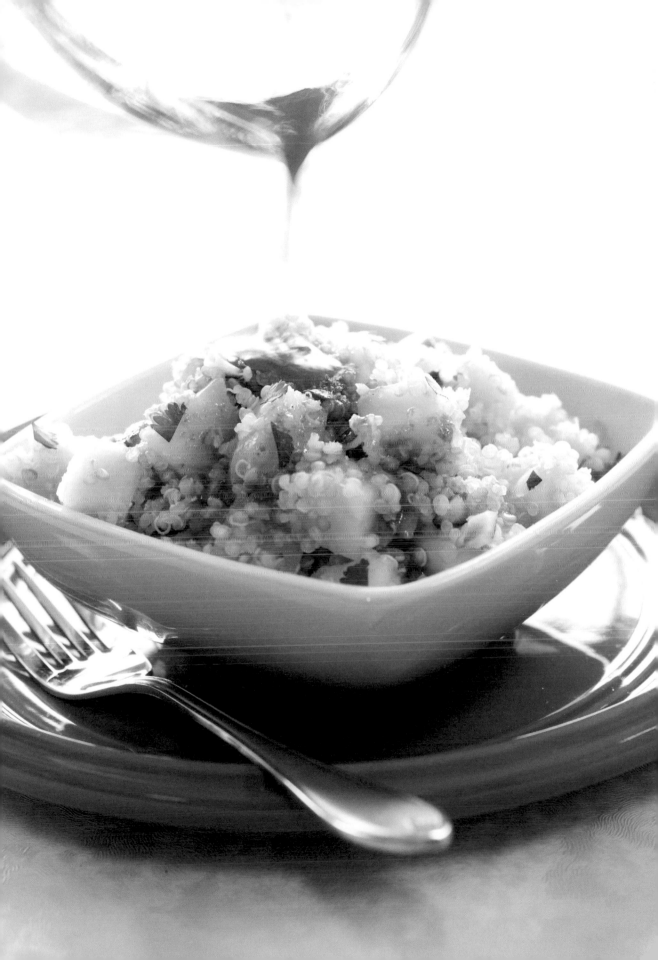

Quinoa

4 servings • PREPARATION: 15 minutes • COOKING TIME: 15 minutes

INGREDIENTS

1 cup (250 ml) uncooked quinoa, rinsed

2½ cups (625 ml) water

1 cup (250 ml) diced fresh pineapple

1 cup (250 ml) diced papaya

½ cup (125 ml) diced mango

½ avocado, peeled and diced

½ cup (125 ml) thinly sliced red onion

1 cup (250 ml) diced cucumber

½ cup (125 ml) finely chopped fresh cilantro or parsley

Freshly ground pepper

For the vinaigrette

Juice of 4 limes or 4 lemons

1 tbsp olive oil

METHOD

In a medium saucepan, combine quinoa and water. Cover and bring to a boil. Reduce heat and simmer for 15 to 20 minutes or until liquid is absorbed. Let cool a little.

In a small bowl, combine ingredients to make vinaigrette.

In a large bowl, combine cooled quinoa, pineapple, papaya, mango, avocado, red onion, cucumber, cilantro and pepper and toss with vinaigrette.

Serve chilled.

Nutrition Facts Per serving	
Amount	% Daily Value
Calories 360	
Fat 10 g	15%
Saturated 1.5 g	8%
+ Trans 0 g	
Polyunsaturated 1.5 g	
Omega-6 1.5 g	
Omega-3 0.1 g	
Monounsaturated 3.5 g	
Cholesterol 0 mg	0%
Sodium 25 mg	1%
Potassium 980 mg	28%
Carbohydrate 58 g	19%
Fiber 10 g	40%
Sugars 14 g	
Protein 9 g	
Vitamin A 91 RE	10%
Vitamin C 114 mg	190%
Calcium 127 mg	10%
Iron 6.7 mg	50%
Phosphorous 248 mg	25%

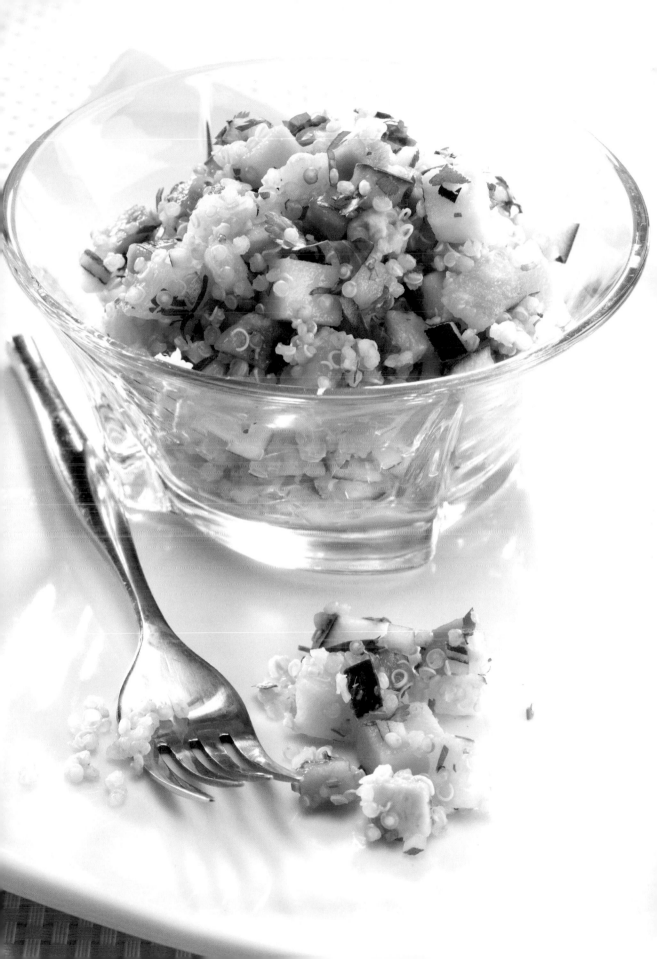

QUINOA
Apple Salad

4 servings • PREPARATION: 15 minutes • COOKING TIME: 20 minutes

INGREDIENTS

1 cup (250 ml) uncooked quinoa, rinsed

2½ cups (625 ml) water

1 bunch mixed greens

1 red pepper, diced

2 apples, cut in pieces

1 cup (250 ml) chopped walnuts

For the vinaigrette

¼ cup (60 ml) olive oil

2 tbsp apple cider vinegar

1 tbsp honey

2 cloves garlic, crushed

2 dates

Pinch ground cinnamon

2 tbsp water

METHOD

In a medium saucepan, combine quinoa and water. Cover and bring to a boil. Reduce heat and simmer for 15 to 20 minutes or until liquid is absorbed. Let cool a little.

In a food processor, mix oil, vinegar, honey, garlic, dates and cinnamon to a smooth purée. Add water as needed to adjust consistency.

Pour vinaigrette into a large bowl.

Add mixed greens, red pepper, apples, walnuts and cooled quinoa. Toss and serve.

Nutrition Facts Per serving	
Amount	**% Daily Value**
Calories 440	
Fat 20 g	31%
Saturated 2 g	10%
+ Trans 0 g	
Polyunsaturated 11 g	
Omega-6 9 g	
Omega-3 2 g	
Monounsaturated 2.5 g	
Cholesterol 0 mg	0%
Sodium 30 mg	1%
Potassium 620 mg	18%
Carbohydrate 55 g	18%
Fiber 7 g	28%
Sugars 15 g	
Protein 11 g	
Vitamin A 190 RE	20%
Vitamin C 50 mg	80%
Calcium 103 mg	10%
Iron 5.7 mg	40%
Phosphorous 291 mg	25%

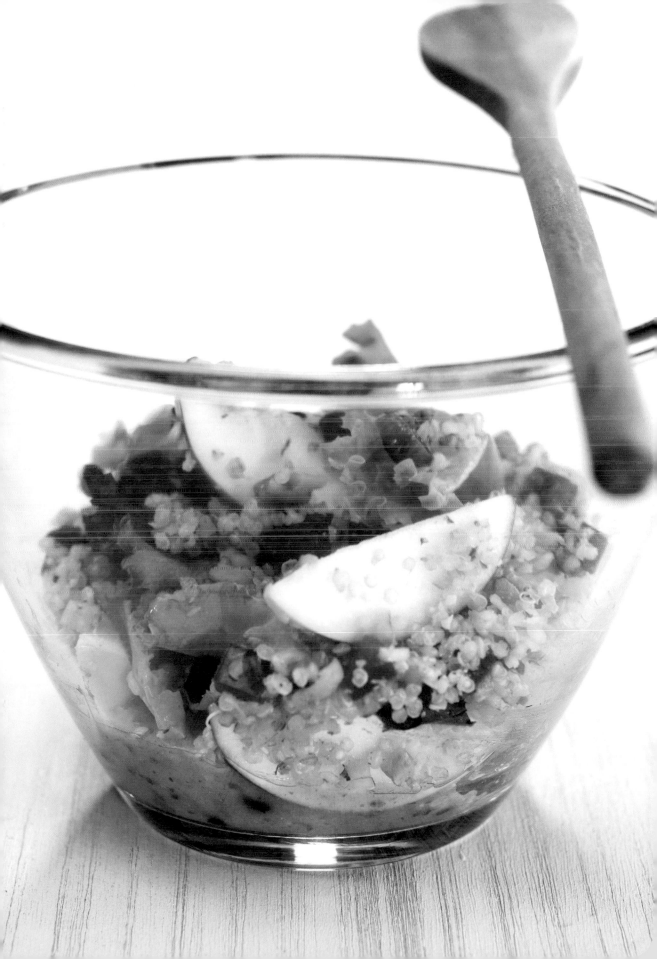

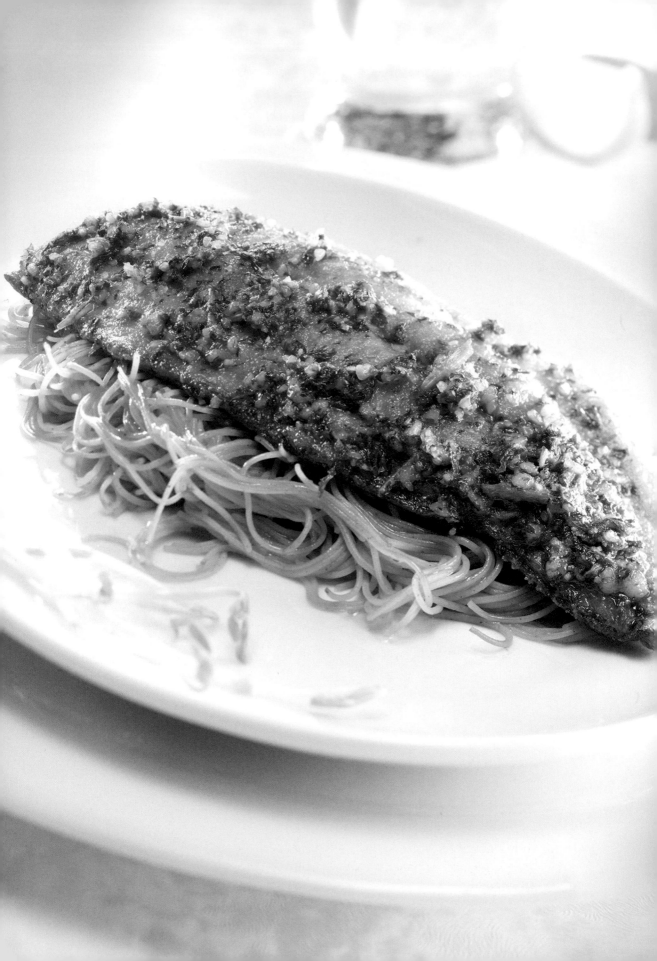

4 servings • PREPARATION: 15 minutes • COOKING TIME: 15 minutes

METHOD

Pesto: In a blender, combine ingredients for pesto and purée.

In a skillet, heat 1 tbsp pesto over medium heat. Add fish and cook, covered, for about 10 minutes or until fish is opaque and flakes easily when tested with a fork.

Once fish is done, add remaining pesto (to avoid destroying the enzymes in the miso, which are sensitive to heat) and reheat gently.

Place fish and pesto on a bed of rice vermicelli.

Serve with Quick and Easy Kale Salad (p. 86).

• • • • • • • • • • • • • •

VARIATION

Use brown rice instead of rice vermicelli.

TIP

You can use any kind of fish rich in omega-3s, such as mackerel, salmon, trout, herring or sardines.

INGREDIENTS

1 lb (454 g) fish (see Tip)

2 cups (500 ml) cooked brown rice vermicelli

For the Pesto

½ cup (125 ml) pine nuts

1 cup (250 ml) fresh spinach, torn in pieces

1 cup (250 ml) fresh basil

1 cup (250 ml) fresh parsley

2 cloves garlic, sliced

1 shallot, sliced

¼ cup (60 ml) olive oil

1 tbsp lemon juice

1 tsp miso, or salt to taste

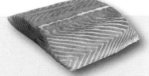

ARTHRITIS INFO

• •

Fish that is rich in omega-3s helps reduce joint stiffness, pain and inflammation in people suffering from arthritis.

Nutrition Facts Per serving	
Amount	% Daily Value
Calories 600	
Fat 30 g	46%
Saturated 5 g	25%
+ Trans 0 g	
Polyunsaturated 7 g	
Omega-6 4.5 g	
Omega-3 3 g	
Monounsaturated 4 g	
Cholesterol 55 mg	18%
Sodium 170 mg	7%
Potassium 750 mg	21%
Carbohydrate 57 g	19%
Fiber 3 g	12%
Sugars 1 g	
Protein 26 g	
Vitamin A 281 RE	30%
Vitamin C 17 mg	30%
Calcium 109 mg	10%
Iron 4.9 mg	35%
Phosphorous 220 mg	20%

SALMON FILLETS
with Anti-Inflammatory Spices

4 servings • PREPARATION: 15 minutes • REFRIGERATION TIME: 3 to 12 hours • COOKING TIME: 10 minutes

INGREDIENTS

1 tbsp paprika

1 tbsp ground cumin

1 tsp coriander seeds

½ tsp red pepper flakes

¼ tsp ground cinnamon

¼ tsp grated fresh ginger

2 tbsp fresh cilantro

½ tsp turmeric

½ tsp salt

Zest of 1 lime, finely chopped

1 small onion, minced

1 clove garlic, very finely chopped

½ cup (125 ml) avocado purée

4 fillets fresh salmon, skinless and boneless (about 1½ lbs/750 g)

METHOD

In a dry nonstick skillet, combine spices and heat over medium heat for 2 minutes. Remove from heat and place in a spice mill or a mortar. Crush to a fine powder and reserve in a bowl.

In a small bowl, combine lime zest, onion, garlic and puréed avocado and add to spice mix.

Place salmon fillets on a dish. Spread spiced avocado purée over each fillet. Refrigerate for 3 to 12 hours.

Preheat oven to 400°F (200°C). Line a baking sheet with parchment paper. Place salmon fillets on prepared baking sheet and bake in preheated oven for 8 minutes or until salmon is cooked.

Serve with rice, vegetables and a salad.

Nutrition Facts Per serving	
Amount	% Daily Value
Calories 260	
Fat 14 g	22%
Saturated 2.5 g	13%
+ Trans 0 g	
Polyunsaturated 4.5 g	
Omega-6 2.5 g	
Omega-3 2 g	
Monounsaturated 6 g	
Cholesterol 60 mg	20%
Sodium 360 mg	15%
Potassium 680 mg	19%
Carbohydrate 12 g	4%
Fiber 3 g	12%
Sugars 2 g	
Protein 22g	
Vitamin A 112 RE	10%
Vitamin C 10 mg	15%
Calcium 78 mg	8%
Iron 2.8 mg	20%
Phosphorous 292 mg	25%

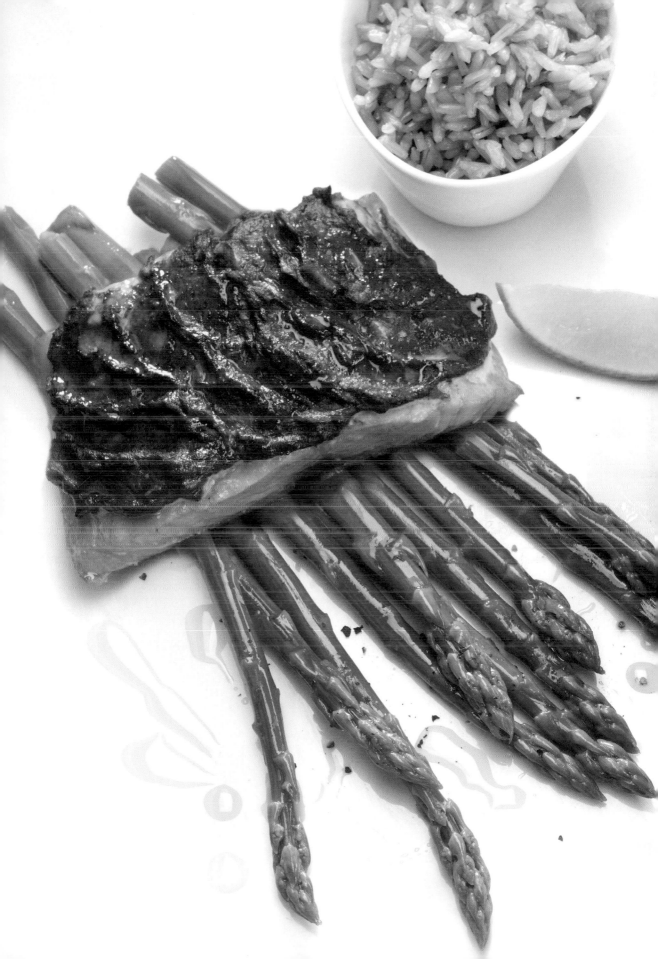

ASIAN TOFU
and Turkey Stir-Fry

4 servings • PREPARATION: 10 minutes • MARINATING TIME: 1 hour • COOKING TIME: 15 minutes

INGREDIENTS

1 block (16 oz/454 g) firm tofu, cut into batonnets

½ lb (225 g) fresh turkey breast, cut into strips

1 carrot, cut into batonnets

1 red, yellow or green pepper, cut into strips

3 stalks celery, sliced thin diagonally

2 cloves garlic, sliced

2 green onions, sliced

2 tsp finely sliced fresh ginger

1 tbsp soy sauce

1 tbsp olive or toasted sesame oil

4 fresh cilantro leaves

Pinch toasted sesame seeds

METHOD

In a large bowl, combine tofu, turkey, carrot, pepper, celery, garlic, onions, ginger and soy sauce. Marinate for 1 hour.

In a skillet, heat oil over medium heat. Add mixture and sauté, stirring occasionally, until turkey is cooked through.

Garnish with cilantro and sesame seeds.

Serve with quinoa or on a bed of rice vermicelli or brown rice.

Nutrition Facts Per serving	
Amount	**% Daily Value**
Calories 230	
Fat 10 g	15%
Saturated 2 g	10%
+ Trans 0 g	
Polyunsaturated 3 g	
Omega-6 2.5 g	
Omega-3 0.3 g	
Monounsaturated 2 g	
Cholesterol 40 mg	13%
Sodium 310 mg	13%
Potassium 630 mg	18%
Carbohydrate 11 g	4%
Fiber 3 g	12%
Sugars 4 g	
Protein 25 g	
Vitamin A 344 RE	35%
Vitamin C 21 mg	35%
Calcium 324 mg	30%
Iron 3.5 mg	25%
Phosphorous 311 mg	30%

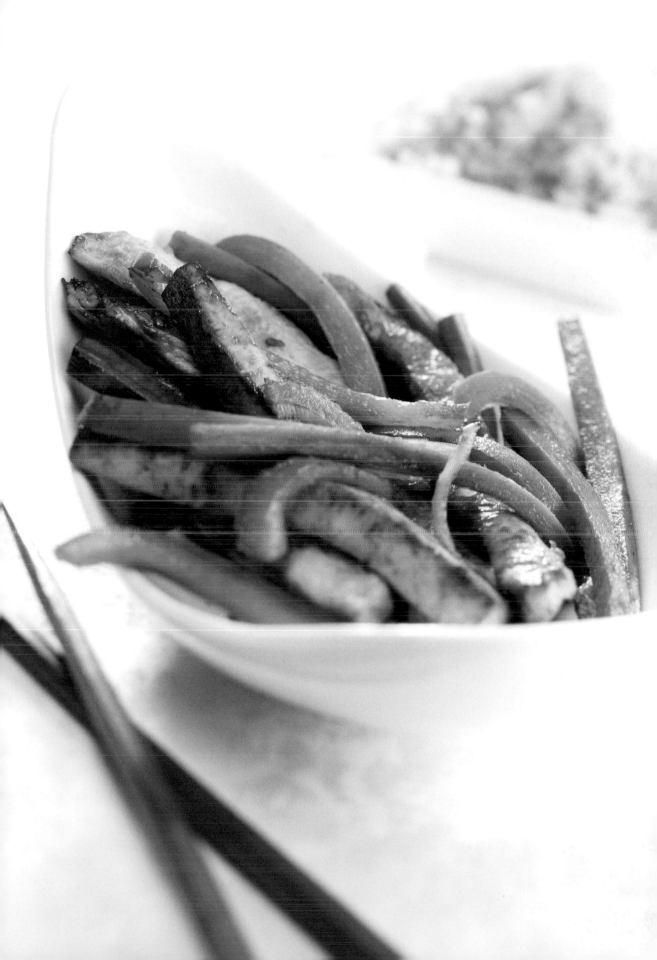

INDIANA
Salmon Cakes

4 servings (8 cakes) • PREPARATION: 30 minutes • COOKING TIME: 15 minutes

INGREDIENTS

1 tbsp olive oil

½ medium onion, finely sliced

1 clove garlic, finely sliced

½ cup (125 ml) diced carrots
or sweet potatoes

1 can (7½ oz/213 g) salmon, drained
(or fresh, skinless and boneless)

2 tbsp sprigs fresh dill

½ cup (125 ml) chopped fresh parsley

½ cup (125 ml) ground chia seeds

4 lemon slices or wedges

METHOD

In a skillet, heat oil over medium-high heat. Add onion, garlic and carrots and sauté until tender. Using a fork, mash to a purée.

Add salmon, dill, parsley and chia seeds. Shape into 8 cakes with your hands.

In a large lightly oiled skillet, brown cakes over medium heat, 4 to 5 minutes per side.

Serve cakes with slices of lemon.

Serve with brown rice or quinoa, and salad or salsa.

Nutrition Facts Per serving	
Amount	**% Daily Value**
Calories 140	
Fat 8 g	12%
Saturated 1 g	5%
+ Trans 0 g	
Polyunsaturated 4 g	
Omega-6 1 g	
Omega-3 3 g	
Monounsaturated 1 g	
Cholesterol 4 mg	2%
Sodium 85 mg	4%
Potassium 160 mg	4%
Carbohydrate 10 g	3%
Fiber 7 g	28%
Sugars 1 g	
Protein 6 g	
Vitamin A 125 RE	15%
Vitamin C 6 mg	10%
Calcium 149 mg	15%
Iron 2.1 mg	15%
Phosphorous 327 mg	30%

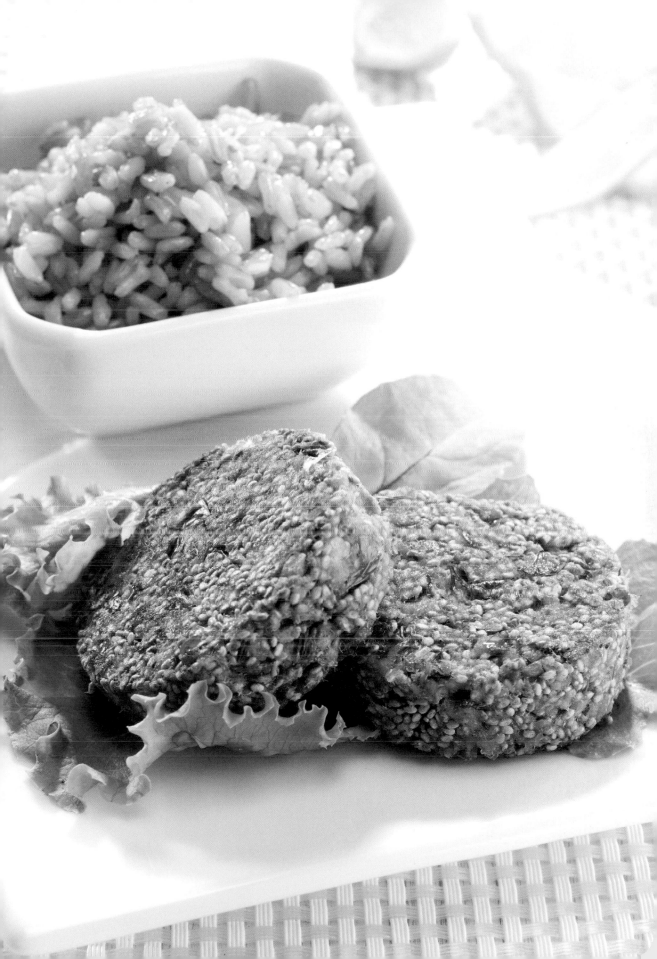

SPRING
Rolls

4 rolls • PREPARATION: 20 minutes

INGREDIENTS

4 round rice paper wrappers (preferably brown)

8 lettuce leaves

⅓ cup (80 ml) Delectable Veggie Pâté (p. 76)

4 slices avocado

1 large green onion, cut into thin strips

8 fresh mint or cilantro leaves

1 cucumber, peeled and julienned

1 rounded tbsp shredded carrot

4 handfuls sprouts, any sort

METHOD

Divide ingredients into four equal parts to make four spring rolls one at a time.

For each roll, submerge a rice paper wrapper in a bowl of lukewarm water to rehydrate. Drain and place on a moist dishtowel.

Place a lettuce leaf in center of rice paper. Spread veggie pâté over it. Top with 1 slice avocado, strips of green onion, 2 mint leaves, cucumber, shredded carrot and 1 handful sprouts, piling ingredients along lettuce leaf. Cover with a second lettuce leaf.

Fold two opposite ends of rice paper wrapper over lettuce and start to roll, making the roll as compact as possible.

Serve with peanut or another sauce, Kale Chips (p. 85), a green salad or brown rice.

Nutrition Facts Per 2 rolls	
Amount	% Daily Value
Calories 260	
Fat 16 g	25%
Saturated 2 g	10%
+ Trans 0 g	
Polyunsaturated 6 g	
Omega-6 10 g	
Omega-3 0.5 g	
Monounsaturated 4.5 g	
Cholesterol 0 mg	0%
Sodium 260 mg	11%
Potassium 980 mg	28%
Carbohydrate 19 g	6%
Fiber 8 g	32%
Sugars 4 g	
Protein 9 g	
Vitamin A 2413 RE	240%
Vitamin C 25 mg	40%
Calcium 156 mg	15%
Iron 5.4 mg	40%
Phosphorous 214 mg	20%

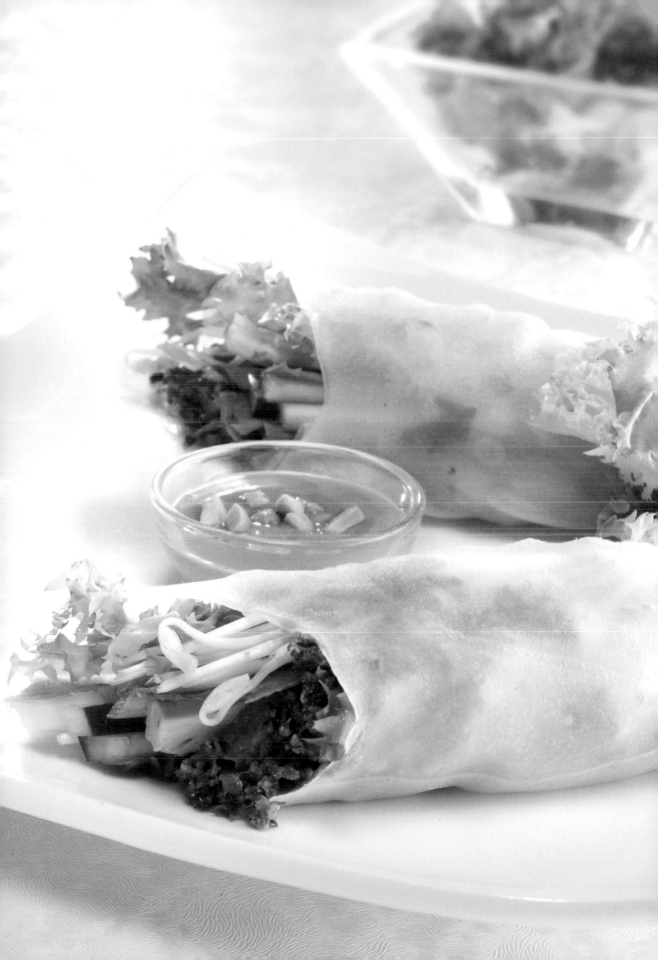

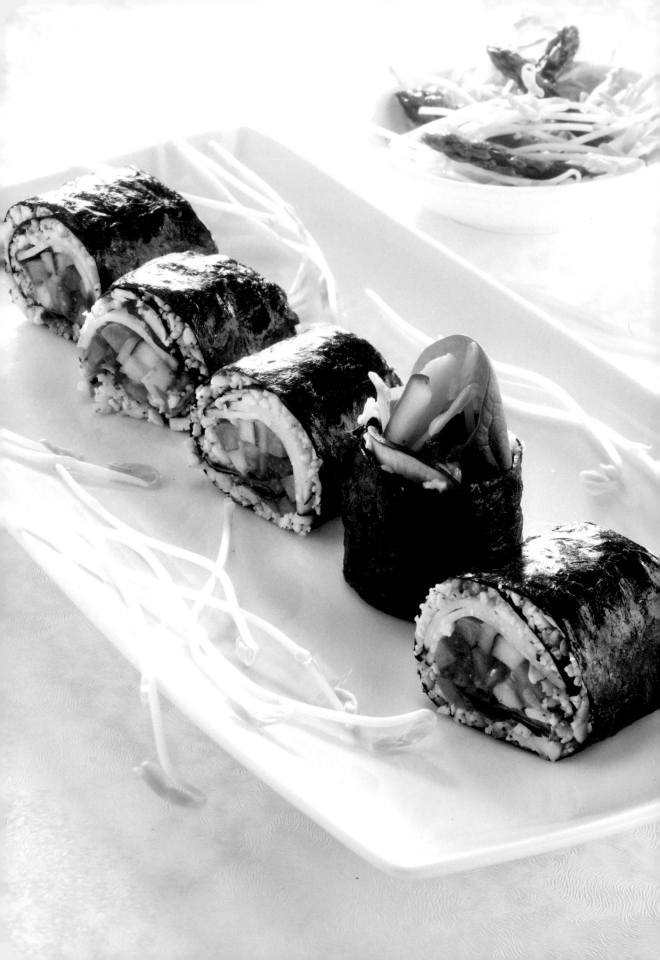

4 servings (approximately 20 makis) • PREPARATION: 15 minutes

METHOD

In a large bowl, combine almond butter and miso. Add crumbled cauliflower and sesame seeds.

Spread mixture equally on nori sheets, leaving a little over 1 inch (2.5 cm) at the top of each sheet to be able to close the roll once filled.

Along center of mixture, place strips of avocado, cucumber, celery, carrot and so on. Add sprouts and herbs. Shape into four tight rolls.

Using a sharp knife, slice each roll into four or six pieces.

Serve with soy or peanut sauce, marinated ginger and wasabi, if desired.

INGREDIENTS

2 tbsp almond or peanut butter

1 tsp miso

2 cups (500 ml) crumbled cauliflower (crumble to the size of grains of rice)

2 tsp toasted sesame seeds

4 sheets nori

2 cups (500 ml) sliced avocado, cucumber, celery, carrots, radishes, spinach, lettuce, strawberries, mango, as desired

Sprouts, to taste

Herbs, to taste

Nutrition Facts Per serving	
Amount	% Daily Value
Calories 80	
Fat 3.5 g	2%
Saturated 0.4 g	2%
+ Trans 0 g	
Polyunsaturated 1 g	
Omega-6 1 g	
Omega-3 0.1 g	
Monounsaturated 2 g	
Cholesterol 0 mg	0%
Sodium 90 mg	4%
Potassium 350 mg	10%
Carbohydrate 8 g	3%
Fiber 3 g	12%
Sugars 2 g	
Protein 4 g	
Vitamin A 50 RE	6%
Vitamin C 69 mg	110%
Calcium 54 mg	4%
Iron 1 mg	8%
Phosphorous 89 mg	8%

TURKEY WITH BASIL PESTO
and Cabbage

4 servings • PREPARATION: 5 minutes • COOKING TIME: 15 to 20 minutes

INGREDIENTS

1 lb (454 g) fresh turkey breast, cut into thin strips

1 clove garlic, sliced

1 onion, sliced

2 cups (500 ml) shredded or thin strips raw cabbage

½ cup (125 ml) vegetable stock

1 tsp miso, or salt to taste

For the basil pesto

1 cup (250 ml) well-packed basil leaves

¼ cup (60 ml) pine nuts

1 tbsp whole chia seeds

¼ cup (60 ml) olive or other oil

1 tsp lemon zest

2 tsp lemon juice

METHOD

Basil pesto: In a food processor, combine basil leaves, pine nuts and chia seeds with olive oil and lemon zest and juice and process until smooth.

In a skillet, sauté turkey strips and a bit of pesto over medium heat for 1 minute.

Add half the pesto, garlic and onion and continue cooking, 4 to 5 minutes. Add remaining pesto, cabbage and stock and continue cooking, covered, 3 or 4 minutes more.

Add miso at the end of cooking and mix well.

Serve with Buckwheat Salad with Pomegranate and Edamame (p. 98) or a green salad.

Nutrition Facts Per serving	
Amount	% Daily Value
Calories 360	
Fat 21 g	32%
Saturated 3 g	15%
+ Trans 0 g	
Polyunsaturated 4 g	
Omega-6 3 g	
Omega-3 1 g	
Monounsaturated 1 g	
Cholesterol 85 mg	28%
Sodium 160 mg	7%
Potassium 660 mg	19%
Carbohydrate 14 g	5%
Fiber 4 g	0%
Sugars 5 g	
Protein 29 g	
Vitamin A 304 RE	30%
Vitamin C 12 mg	20%
Calcium 117 mg	10%
Iron 3.2 mg	25%
Phosphorous 313 mg	30%

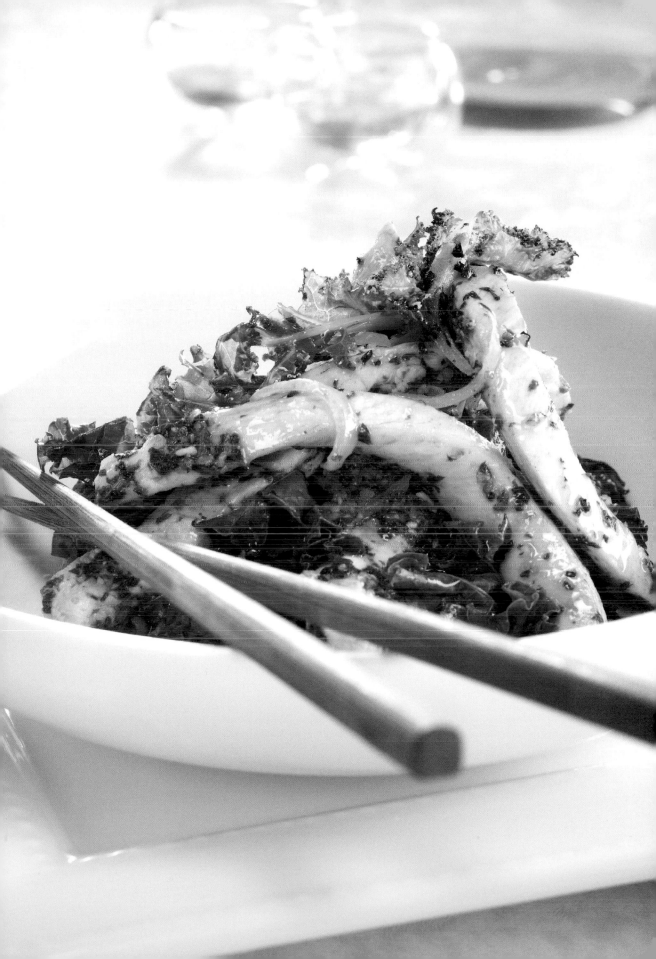

FIESTA VEGETABLE
Frittata

4 servings • PREPARATION: 10 minutes • COOKING TIME: 15 minutes

INGREDIENTS

1 tbsp olive or other oil

1 onion, sliced

1 clove garlic, sliced

½ cup (125 ml) mushrooms, sliced

1 stalk celery, sliced thin diagonally

¼ cup (60 ml) water

8 eggs, beaten

½ tomato, diced

1 cup (250 ml) torn spinach
or 1 cup (250 ml) kale

2 tsp fresh thyme

Freshly ground pepper

2 tbsp salsa

METHOD

Preheat the oven to 350°F (180°C).

In a skillet, heat oil over medium heat and sauté onion, garlic, mushrooms and celery.

In a bowl, combine remaining ingredients, except for the salsa.

Transfer mixture to skillet and continue cooking for 6 minutes.

Place frittata in preheated oven and continue cooking for 4 minutes. Serve with salsa.

Serve with a salad or rice and raw vegetables for a main course, or with fruit for breakfast.

Nutrition Facts Per serving		
Amount		% Daily Value
Calories 210		
Fat 13 g		20%
Saturated 3.5 g		18%
+ Trans 0 g		
Polyunsaturated 1.5 g		
Omega-6 1.5 g		
Omega-3 0.1 g		
Monounsaturated 4.5 g		
Cholesterol 370 mg		123%
Sodium 190 mg		8%
Potassium 330 mg		9%
Carbohydrate 330 g		9%
Fiber 8 g		3%
Sugars 3 g		
Protein 14 g		
Vitamin A 189 RE		20%
Vitamin C 4 mg		6%
Calcium 84 mg		8%
Iron 1.6 mg		10%
Phosphorous 170 mg		15%

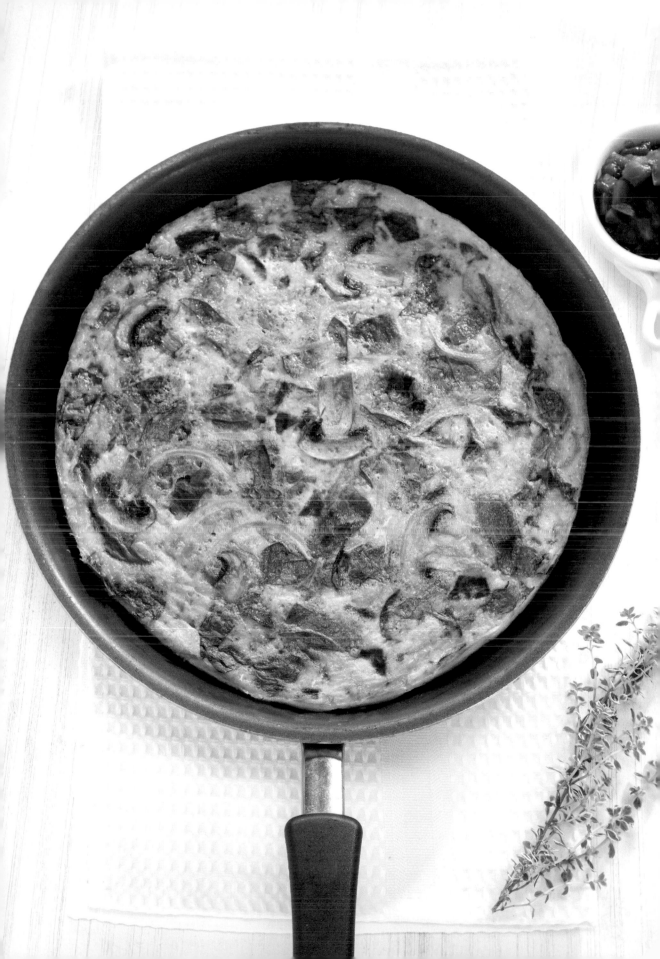

CHICKEN
with Mango Salsa

4 servings • PREPARATION: 15 minutes • COOKING TIME: 10 minutes

INGREDIENTS

1 tbsp olive oil

1 onion, finely sliced

1 clove garlic, finely sliced

1 lb (454 g) boneless, skinless chicken breast, diced

For the Mango Salsa

1 mango, cut in small pieces

1 tsp lime or lemon zest

1 tbsp lime or lemon juice

1 tsp honey or maple syrup

1 tbsp chopped fresh cilantro

1 tsp miso

Freshly ground pepper

METHOD

Mango salsa: In a bowl, combine mango, lime zest and juice, honey or maple syrup, cilantro, miso and pepper. Let stand for about 10 minutes.

Meanwhile, heat oil in a skillet over medium heat and sauté onion, garlic and chicken, 3 to 4 minutes until chicken is no longer pink inside.

In a saucepan over low heat, gently heat salsa (not too hot because the miso contains enzymes that are sensitive to heat). Pour over chicken.

Serve with rice vermicelli or quinoa and a salad.

Nutrition Facts Per serving	
Amount	% Daily Value
Calories 240	
Fat 7 g	11%
Saturated 1.5 g	8%
+ Trans 0 g	
Polyunsaturated 1 g	
Omega-6 1 g	
Omega-3 0.1 g	
Monounsaturated 1 g	
Cholesterol 80 mg	27%
Sodium 150 mg	6%
Potassium 450 mg	13%
Carbohydrate 17 g	6%
Fiber 2 g	8%
Sugars 11 g	
Protein 26 g	
Vitamin A 61 RE	6%
Vitamin C 13 mg	20%
Calcium 47 mg	4%
Iron 1.5 mg	10%
Phosphorous 226 mg	20%

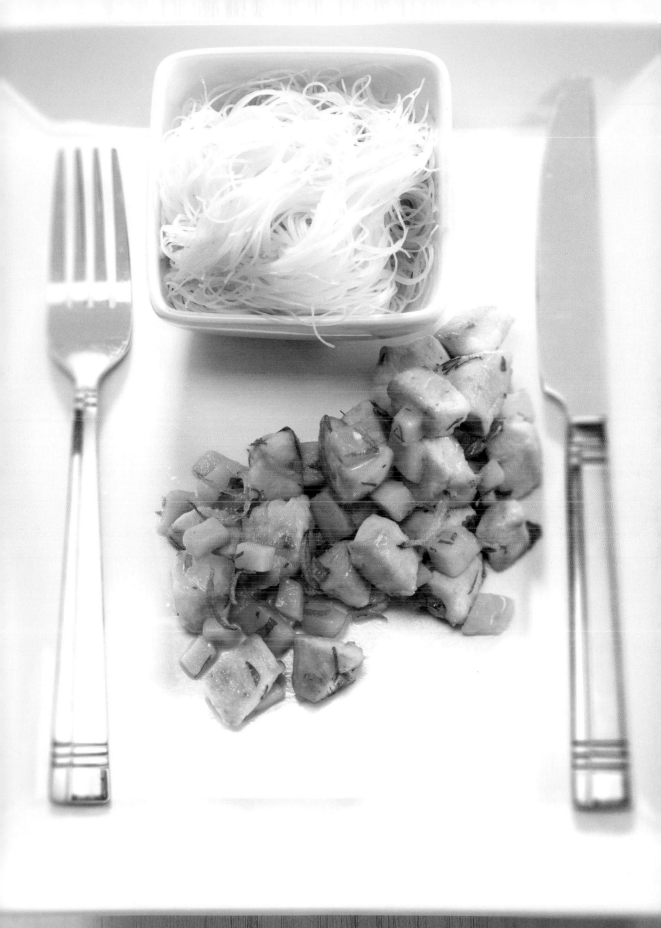

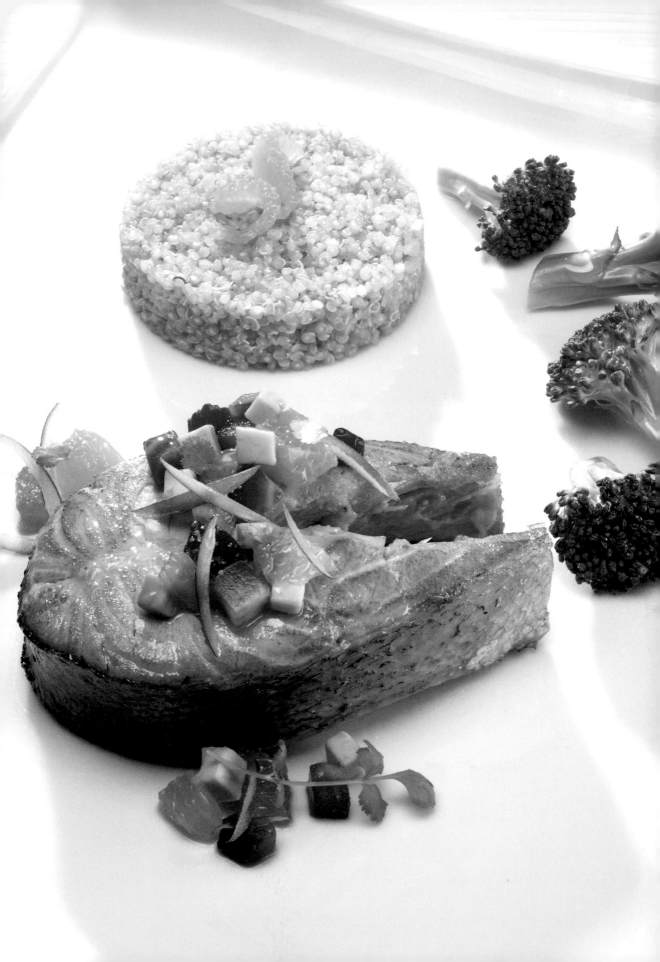

SALMON WITH AVOCADO
and Citrus Salsa

4 servings • PREPARATION: 15 minutes • COOKING TIME: 10 minutes

METHOD

In a skillet, heat oil over medium-high heat and sauté garlic and shallot.

Add salmon steaks and cook about 3 minutes per side or until salmon is cooked through.

Avocado and citrus salsa: In a large bowl, combine ingredients for salsa.

Serve salmon with salsa.

Serve on a bed of quinoa or rice, if desired, and with vegetables (broccoli, Brussels sprouts) or a salad.

INGREDIENTS

1 tbsp olive or other oil

1 clove garlic, sliced

1 shallot, sliced

4 fresh salmon steaks, each about 5 oz (150 g)

For the Avocado and Citrus Salsa

1 avocado, diced

4 strawberries, diced

½ orange, diced

1 pink grapefruit, diced

2 tbsp sliced red onion

2 tbsp chopped fresh cilantro

Pinch Espelette or cayenne pepper

1 tbsp miso

Nutrition Facts Per serving	
Amount	**% Daily Value**
Calories 350	
Fat 17 g	26%
Saturated 3 g	15%
+ Trans 0 g	
Polyunsaturated 3 g	
Omega-6 1 g	
Omega-3 1.5 g	
Monounsaturated 7 g	
Cholesterol 60 mg	20%
Sodium 200 mg	8%
Potassium 940 mg	27%
Carbohydrate 11 g	4%
Fiber 4 g	16%
Sugars 3 g	
Protein 37 g	
Vitamin A 65 RE	6%
Vitamin C 14 mg	25%
Calcium 107 mg	10%
Iron 1.8 mg	15%
Phosphorous 1134 mg	100%

EASY PEASY INDIAN
Chicken

4 servings • PREPARATION: 15 minutes • COOKING TIME: 1 hour

INGREDIENTS

1 tbsp olive oil

1 lb (454 g) boneless skinless chicken breasts

1 red onion, finely chopped

1 clove garlic, sliced

1 red pepper, cut in pieces

1 green pepper, cut in pieces

1 stalk celery, cut in pieces

1 cup (250 ml) chickpeas, cooked

1 tsp ground cumin

1 tsp turmeric

1 tsp curry powder

2 tsp chopped fresh ginger

¾ cup (180 ml) almond milk

Miso, to taste

Freshly ground pepper

METHOD

Preheat oven to 400°F (200°C).

Lightly grease an ovenproof dish.

In a skillet, heat oil over medium heat and lightly sauté chicken with onion, garlic, peppers and celery. Transfer to prepared ovenproof dish.

Add remaining ingredients (except miso and pepper). Cover with aluminum foil and bake in preheated oven for 1 hour.

Right before serving, add miso, season and mix well.

Serve with vegetables or on a bed of basmati rice or quinoa.

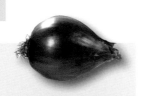

ARTHRITIS INFO

• •

Red onions contain quercetin, a flavonoid with powerful antioxidant properties. It may help fight joint inflammation. Red and yellow varieties are good sources of quercetin, as are apples, broccoli, red grapes, cherries, citrus fruit, berries, tea and red wine.

Nutrition Facts Per serving	
Amount	% Daily Value
Calories 280	
Fat 7 g	11%
Saturated 1 g	5%
+ Trans 0 g	
Polyunsaturated 1 g	
Omega-6 1 g	
Omega-3 0.1 g	
Monounsaturated 1 g	
Cholesterol 65 mg	22%
Sodium 160 mg	6%
Potassium 800 mg	23%
Carbohydrate 24 g	8%
Fiber 5 g	20%
Sugars 7 g	
Protein 31 g	
Vitamin A 92 RE	10%
Vitamin C 38 mg	60%
Calcium 85 mg	8%
Iron 3.6 mg	25%
Phosphorous 379 mg	35%

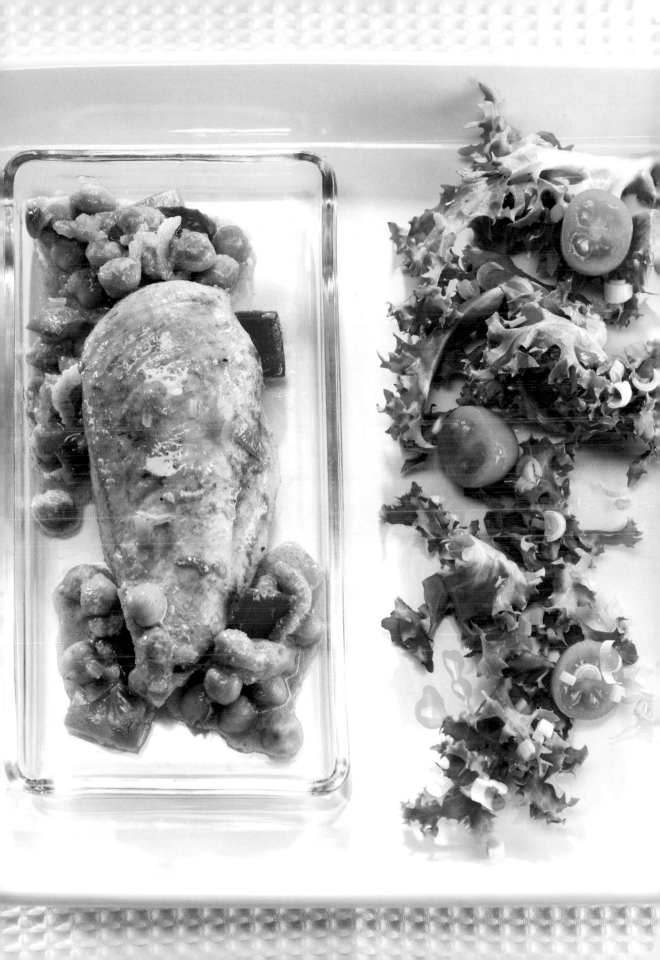

RICE VERMICELLI WITH SALMON
and Ginger

4 servings • PREPARATION: 10 minutes • COOKING TIME: 10 minutes

INGREDIENTS

1 tbsp olive or other oil

2 green onions, sliced

1 clove garlic, sliced

1 red pepper, cut into strips

1 stalk celery, sliced diagonally

2 cups (500 ml) broccoli florets

½ cup (125 ml) orange juice
or 1 peeled orange, finely chopped

1 tsp grated fresh ginger

1 lb (454 g) fresh skinless salmon, diced

1 tsp miso

3 tbsp water

Freshly ground pepper

2 cups (500 ml) cooked brown rice vermicelli

METHOD

In a skillet, heat oil over medium heat and sauté vegetables, about 5 minutes.

Add orange juice or chopped orange, ginger and salmon and continue cooking, 3 or 4 minutes. Add miso and water. Season with pepper to taste, and serve over rice vermicelli.

• • • • • • • • • • • • • •

VARIATION

Try soba noodles instead of rice vermicelli.

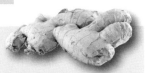

ARTHRITIS INFO

Studies show that people suffering from rheumatoid arthritis who eat ginger regularly experience less pain, stiffness and inflammation. To feel relief, it takes only a single ¼-inch (5 mm) slice of ginger daily. Fresh ginger is the most effective form.

Nutrition Facts Per serving	
Amount	% Daily Value
Calories 440	
Fat 11 g	17%
Saturated 2 g	8%
+ Trans 0 g	
Polyunsaturated 3 g	
Omega-6 0.5 g	
Omega-3 2.5 g	
Monounsaturated 2.5 g	
Cholesterol 60 mg	20%
Sodium 135 mg	6%
Potassium 910 mg	26%
Carbohydrate 60 g	20%
Fiber 3 g	12%
Sugars 5 g	
Protein 25 g	
Vitamin A 129 RE	15%
Vitamin C 50 mg	80%
Calcium 71 mg	6%
Iron 3.3 mg	25%
Phosphorous 288 mg	25%

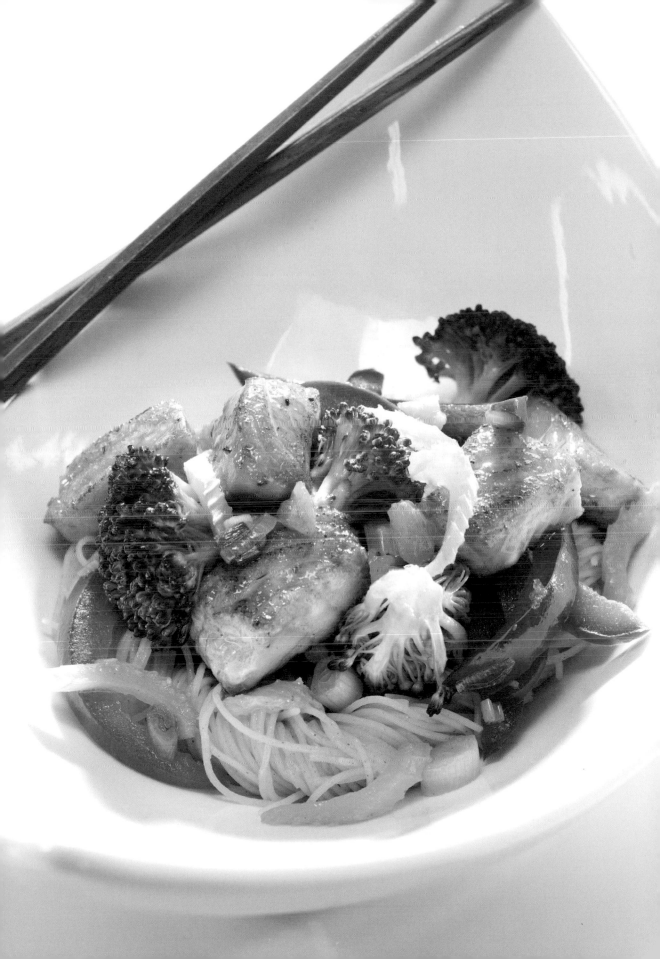

FISH FILLETS
with Fines Herbes

4 servings • PREPARATION: 10 minutes • COOKING TIME: 10 minutes

INGREDIENTS

1 tsp dried basil

1 tsp dried thyme

1 tsp dried rosemary

½ tsp salt

½ tsp freshly ground pepper

4 fish fillets (about 1½ lbs/680 g)
(see Tip)

2 tomatoes, halved

2 tsp olive oil

1 lemon, quartered

METHOD

In a small bowl, combine herbs and spices.

Rub half the spice mixture on fish fillets. Sprinkle remaining on inside of tomato halves.

In a skillet, heat oil over medium-high heat. Add fish fillets and cook, about 4 minutes.

Turn fish and add tomatoes. Cook for 6 minutes or until fish flakes easily when tested with a fork. Turn tomatoes halfway through cooking.

Garnish with lemon quarters.

Serve with quinoa, brown rice vermicelli or brown rice and a vegetable such as broccoli.

• • • • • • • • • • • • • •

TIP

You can use salmon, mackerel, halibut, herring or sardines.

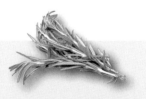

ARTHRITIS INFO

• •

Rosemary has rosmarinic acid, a plant-based polyphenol in the form of extracts that can help relieve symptoms of rheumatoid arthritis. This acid also has antioxidant and anti-inflammatory properties that help reduce inflammation.

Nutrition Facts Per serving		
Amount		% Daily Value
Calories 260		
Fat 13 g		20%
Saturated 2 g		10%
+ Trans 0 g		
Polyunsaturated 4.5 g		
Omega-6 1 g		
Omega-3 3.5 g		
Monounsaturated 3.5 g		
Cholesterol 95 mg		32%
Sodium 370 mg		15%
Potassium 880 mg		25%
Carbohydrate 2 g		1%
Fiber 1 g		4%
Sugars 0 g		
Protein 34 g		
Vitamin A 31 RE		4%
Vitamin C 4 mg		6%
Calcium 37 mg		4%
Iron 2 mg		15%
Phosphorous 346 mg		30%

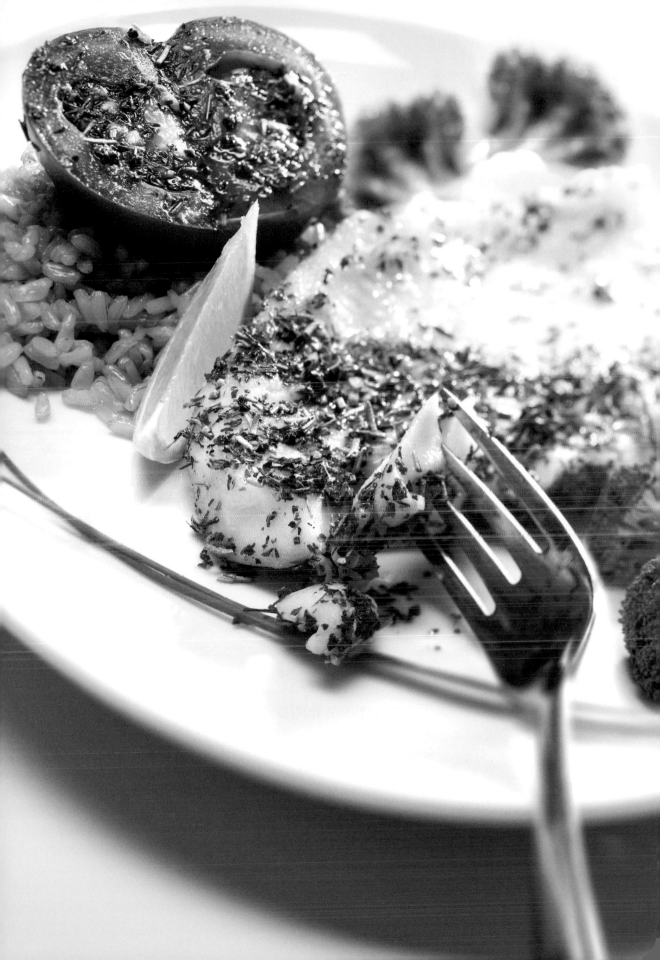

FISH
en Papillote

4 servings (4 papillotes) • PREPARATION: 10 minutes • COOKING TIME: 20 minutes

INGREDIENTS

4 fish fillets (around 1½ lbs/750 g) (see Tip)

1 tbsp lemon juice

1 clove garlic, sliced

1 shallot, sliced

Pinch fresh chopped basil

Freshly ground pepper and salt, or salt substitute, to taste

1 stalk celery, chopped

½ red pepper, cut into small pieces

4 tomatoes, sliced

4 lemons, sliced

METHOD

Preheat oven to 325°F (160°C).

Place each of the fillets on aluminum foil.

In a bowl, combine lemon juice, garlic, shallot, basil and seasoning. Add celery, pepper, tomatoes and lemons.

Divide seasoned vegetable mixture and place on fish fillets. Fold aluminum foil to form packets.

Bake in preheated oven, about 20 minutes.

Serve with salad.

• • • • • • • • • • • • • •

TIP

You can use salmon, mackerel, halibut, herring or sardines.

Nutrition Facts Per serving	
Amount	**% Daily Value**
Calories 240	
Fat 9 g	14%
Saturated 2.5 g	13%
+ Trans 0 g	
Polyunsaturated 2.5 g	
Omega-6 0.3 g	
Omega-3 2 g	
Monounsaturated 3 g	
Cholesterol 55 mg	18%
Sodium 115 mg	5%
Potassium 780 mg	22%
Carbohydrate 15 g	5%
Fiber 4 g	16%
Sugars 4 g	
Protein 25 g	
Vitamin A 92 RE	10%
Vitamin C 36 mg	60%
Calcium 76 mg	6%
Iron 2.3 mg	15%
Phosphorous 188 mg	15%

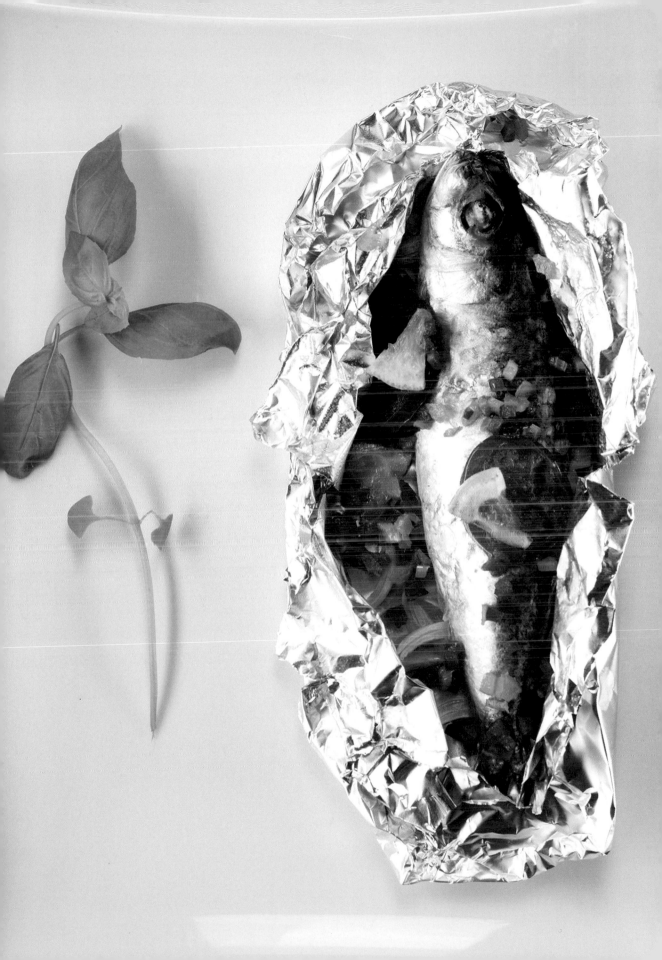

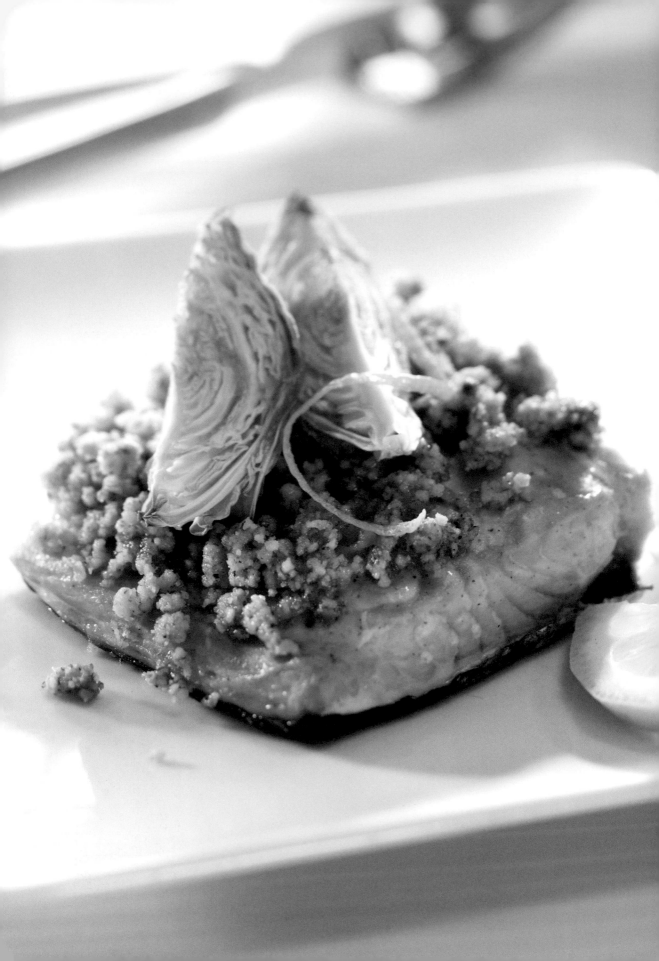

NUT-CRUSTED
Salmon

4 servings • PREPARATION: 5 minutes • REFRIGERATION TIME: 30 minutes • COOKING TIME: 25 minutes

METHOD

Preheat the oven to 350°F (180°C).

In a food processor or with a hand blender, crush walnuts, orange zest and ginger. Add 2 tbsp olive oil and mix to a paste.

Brush salmon fillets with mustard. Divide walnut mixture among fillets. Refrigerate at least 30 minutes.

Line a baking sheet with parchment paper. Combine Brussels sprouts with remaining olive oil and place around edge of a baking sheet.

Bake Brussels sprouts in preheated oven, for 12 minutes.

Place dressed fillets in center of baking sheet and cook for 10 to 15 minutes more.

Serve with quartered lemon.

INGREDIENTS

¾ cup (180 ml) walnuts

Zest of 1 orange

1 tsp ground ginger

3 tbsp extra virgin olive oil, divided

4 salmon fillets (1½ lbs/750 g approx. total)

2 tbsp Dijon mustard

2 cups (500 ml) Brussels sprouts, halved

1 lemon, quartered

Nutrition Facts
Per serving

Amount	% Daily Value
Calories 480	
Fat 33 g	51%
Saturated 4 g	20%
+ Trans 0 g	
Polyunsaturated 15 g	
Omega-6 10 g	
Omega-3 5 g	
Monounsaturated 12 g	
Cholesterol 85 mg	28%
Sodium 160 mg	7%
Potassium 1060 mg	30%
Carbohydrate 10 g	3%
Fiber 4 g	16%
Sugars 2 g	
Protein 35 g	
Vitamin A 58 RE	6%
Vitamin C 27 mg	45%
Calcium 73 mg	6%
Iron 2.9 mg	20%
Phosphorous 410 mg	35%

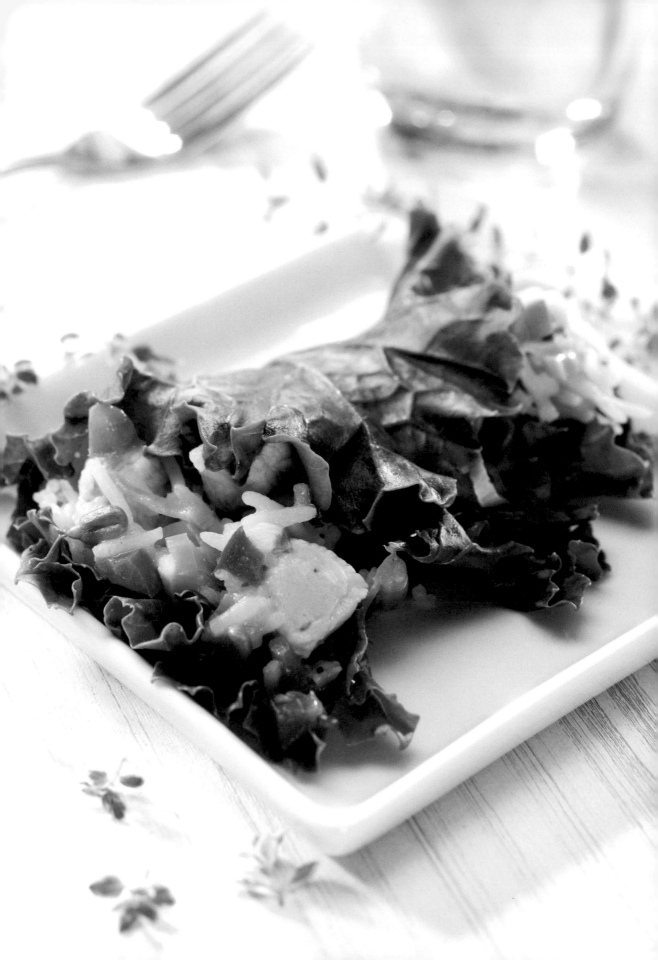

KALE STUFFED WITH POULTRY
and Basmati Rice

6 servings • PREPARATION: 15 minutes • COOKING TIME: 20-30 minutes

METHOD

Steam kale for about 2 minutes until tender.

In a saucepan, heat olive oil over high heat and sauté red pepper and leek for 1 minute.

Add rice and sunflower seeds, stirring, for 1 minute. Add water, thyme, rosemary, cumin and pepper and simmer for 10 to 15 minutes or until rice is cooked. Add poultry and stir to combine.

Divide mixture onto kale leaves. Fold leaves to form rolls.

Serve stuffed kale right away or reheat in a 375°F (190°C) oven for a few minutes.

INGREDIENTS

6 kale leaves

1 tbsp olive oil

1 red pepper, diced

1 leek, sliced

1½ cups (375 ml) uncooked basmati rice

¼ cup (60 ml) sunflower seeds

3 cups (750 ml) water

3 sprigs thyme

¼ tsp dried rosemary

½ tsp ground cumin

Freshly ground pepper

1 lb (454 g) chicken or turkey breast, cooked and diced

Nutrition Facts
Per serving

Amount	% Daily Value
Calories 300	
Fat 8 g	12%
Saturated 1.5 g	8%
+ Trans 0 g	
Polyunsaturated 2.5 g	
Omega-6 2 g	
Omega-3 0 g	
Monounsaturated 0.5 g	
Cholesterol 0 mg	0%
Sodium 10 mg	0%
Potassium 90 mg	3%
Carbohydrate 50 g	17%
Fiber 4 g	16%
Sugars 2 g	
Protein 6 g	
Vitamin A 49 RE	4%
Vitamin C 14 mg	25%
Calcium 28 mg	2%
Iron 2.4 mg	15%
Phosphorous 78 mg	8%

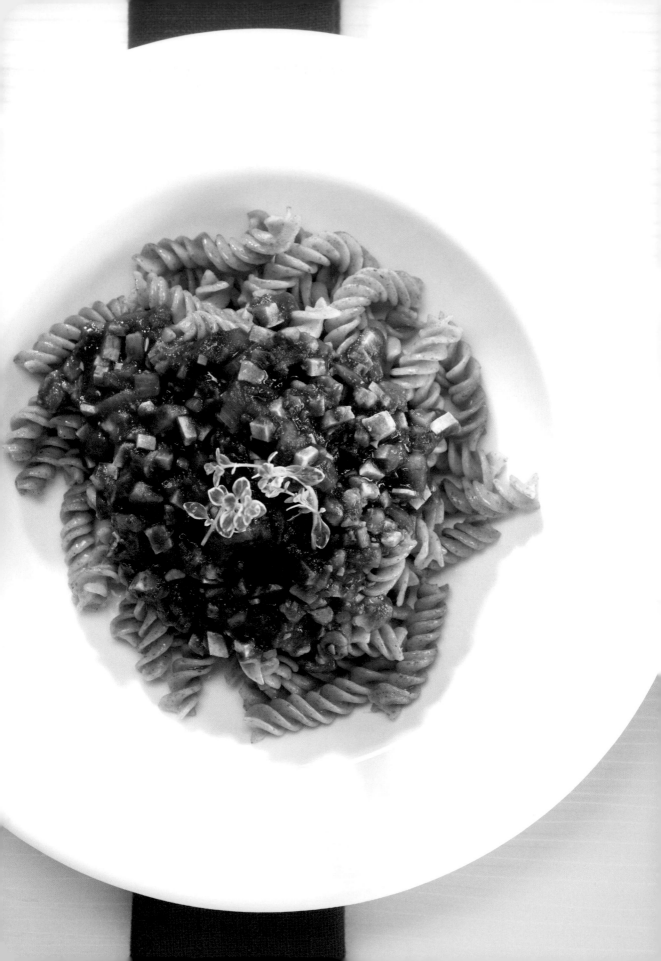

MEATLESS BOLOGNESE
Sauce

6 servings • PREPARATION: 10 minutes • COOKING TIME: 45 minutes

METHOD

In a saucepan, heat olive oil over medium heat and sauté onion and garlic, stirring constantly, for 2 minutes.

Add remaining ingredients, except miso. Reduce heat to low and cook, covered, stirring occasionally, for 40 minutes. Add miso at the end of cooking to protect the enzymes.

Serve over wholewheat pasta or brown rice.

INGREDIENTS

1 tbsp olive oil

1 onion, finely chopped

2 cloves garlic, chopped

1 jar (28 oz/796 ml) tomato sauce

1 cup (250 ml) finely chopped eggplant

1 cup (250 ml) finely chopped mushrooms

⅔ cup (160 ml) finely chopped firm tofu

½ cup (125 ml) finely chopped walnuts

1 tbsp dried oregano

2 tsp dried thyme

Pinch ground cinnamon

1 tsp miso

Nutrition Facts Per serving	
Amount	% Daily Value
Calories 170	
Fat 8 g	12%
Saturated 1 g	5%
+ Trans 0 g	
Polyunsaturated 4 g	
Omega-6 3 g	
Omega-3 0.5 g	
Monounsaturated 1 g	
Cholesterol 0 mg	0%
Sodium 760 mg	32%
Potassium 680 mg	19%
Carbohydrate 19 g	6%
Fiber 4 g	16%
Sugars 8 g	
Protein 6 g	
Vitamin A 59 RE	6%
Vitamin C 7 mg	10%
Calcium 110 mg	10%
Iron 3 mg	20%
Phosphorous 124 mg	10%

SUMMER FRUIT SALAD
with Chia Seeds

4 servings • PREPARATION: 15 minutes

INGREDIENTS

¼ cup (60 ml) fresh raspberries

¼ cup (60 ml) diced pineapple

¼ cup (60 ml) diced papaya

½ cup (125 ml) diced mango

1 tbsp whole chia seeds

2 tbsp water

1 tbsp maple syrup or honey (optional)

4 mint leaves

METHOD

In a bowl, combine fruit, chia seeds, water, and maple syrup or honey, if desired.

Divide fruit salad into four dessert cups.

Garnish each with a mint leaf.

Nutrition Facts
Per serving

Amount	% Daily Value
Calories 70	
Fat 1.5 g	2%
Saturated 0.1 g	1%
+ Trans 0 g	
Polyunsaturated 1 g	
Omega-6 0.3 g	
Omega-3 0.5 g	
Monounsaturated 0.1 g	
Cholesterol 0 mg	0%
Sodium 3 mg	0%
Potassium 100 mg	3%
Carbohydrate 12 g	4%
Fiber 3 g	12%
Sugars 8 g	
Protein 1 g	
Vitamin A 47 RE	4%
Vitamin C 19 mg	30%
Calcium 39 mg	4%
Iron 0.7 mg	4%
Phosphorous 43 mg	4%

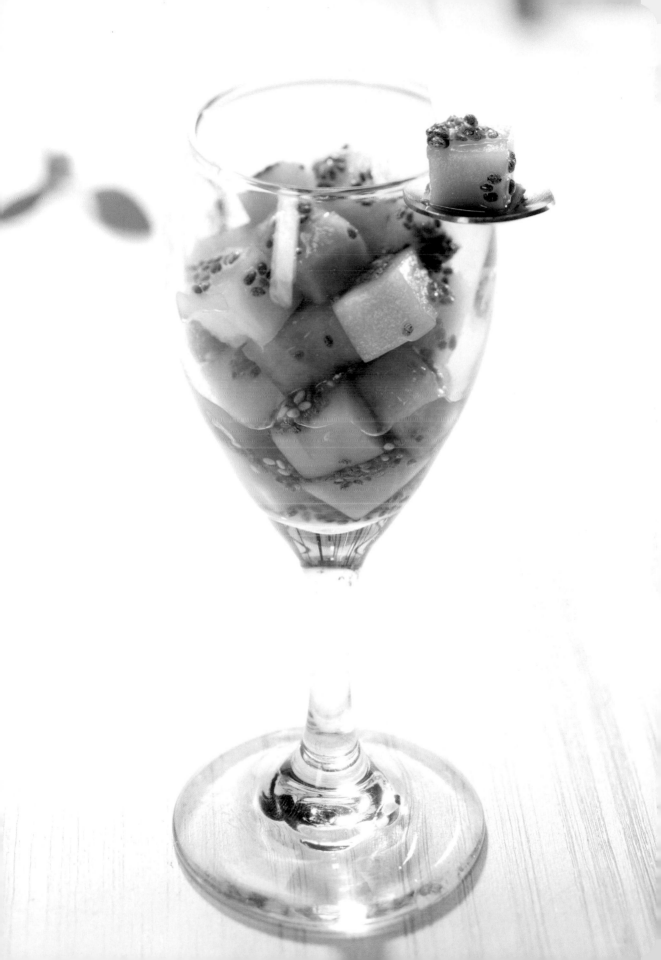

Quinoa Drops

14 drop cookies • PREPARATION: 15 minutes • COOKING TIME: 7 minutes

INGREDIENTS

½ cup (125 ml) cooked quinoa

½ cup (125 ml) walnuts

1 cup (250 ml) finely chopped dates

½ cup (125 ml) applesauce

1 egg

2 tbsp buckwheat flour

METHOD

Preheat oven to 275°F (140°C).

In a food processor, crush quinoa with walnuts.

In a bowl, using a whisk, mix chopped dates with applesauce and egg. Add quinoa and nut mixture and buckwheat flour. Combine.

Line a baking sheet with parchment paper. Shape mixture into approximately 14 small balls and place on prepared baking sheet. Bake in preheated oven on middle rack of oven, 6 to 7 minutes. Cool before serving.

Nutrition Facts
Per quinoa drop

Amount	% Daily Value
Calories 100	
Fat 3 g	5%
Saturated 0.3 g	2%
+ Trans 0 g	
Polyunsaturated 1.5 g	
Omega-6 1.5 g	
Omega-3 0.3 g	
Monounsaturated 0.5 g	
Cholesterol 15 mg	5%
Sodium 5 mg	0%
Potassium 170 mg	5%
Carbohydrate 17 g	6%
Fiber 2 g	8%
Sugars 10 g	
Protein 2 g	
Vitamin A 5 RE	0%
Vitamin C 1 mg	2%
Calcium 15 mg	2%
Iron 0.9 mg	6%
Phosphorous 54 mg	4%

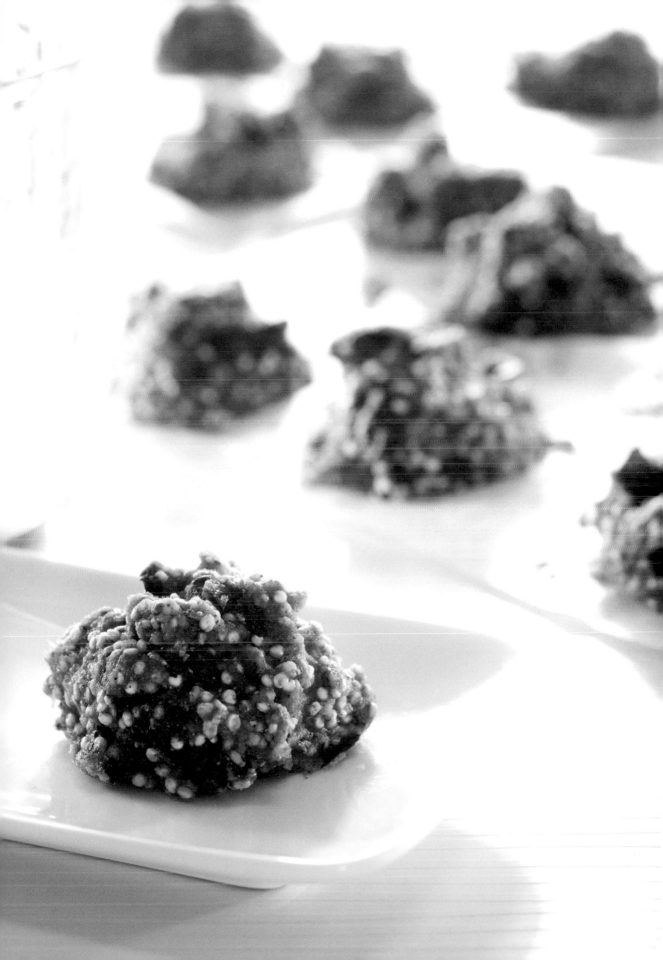

Cinnamon Apple Crisp

8 servings (1 large pie plate) • PREPARATION: 15 minutes

INGREDIENTS

1 cup (250 ml) almonds, ground

½ cup (125 ml) pecans
or hazelnuts, coarsely chopped

2 tbsp chia seeds, ground

½ cup (125 ml) dates, finely
chopped, divided

2 tbsp flaxseeds, finely ground
(with a coffee grinder)

1 tsp ground cinnamon
(or more, to taste)

4 apples, diced, plus 1 apple,
sliced and brushed with lemon juice
(for garnish)

1 tsp lemon juice

¼ cup (60 ml) pecans, chopped

Pinch ground cinnamon

2 tbsp maple syrup (optional)

METHOD

Grind almonds, ½ cup (125 ml) pecans or hazelnuts, chia seeds and ¼ cup (60 ml) dates. Place mixture in a pie plate and flatten with your fingers. Add water as needed, lining the bottom of the pie plate with the mixture. Refrigerate while you prepare the apple filling.

For the apple filling, mix flaxseeds, remaining dates, 1 tsp cinnamon, diced apples and lemon juice. Pour filling over crust.

Top with ¼ cup (60 ml) chopped pecans, apple slices, a pinch of cinnamon and a drizzle of maple syrup, if desired.

Serve chilled or at room temperature.

Nutrition Facts Per serving	
Amount	**% Daily Value**
Calories 210	
Fat 10 g	15%
Saturated 1 g	5%
+ Trans 0 g	
Polyunsaturated 3.5 g	
Omega-6 2.5 g	
Omega-3 1 g	
Monounsaturated 4.5 g	
Cholesterol 0 mg	0%
Sodium 45 mg	2%
Potassium 240 mg	7%
Carbohydrate 28 g	9%
Fiber 6 g	24%
Sugars 20 g	
Protein 2 g	
Vitamin A 6 RE	0%
Vitamin C 5 mg	8%
Calcium 53 mg	4%
Iron 1.5 mg	8%
Phosphorous 85 mg	8%

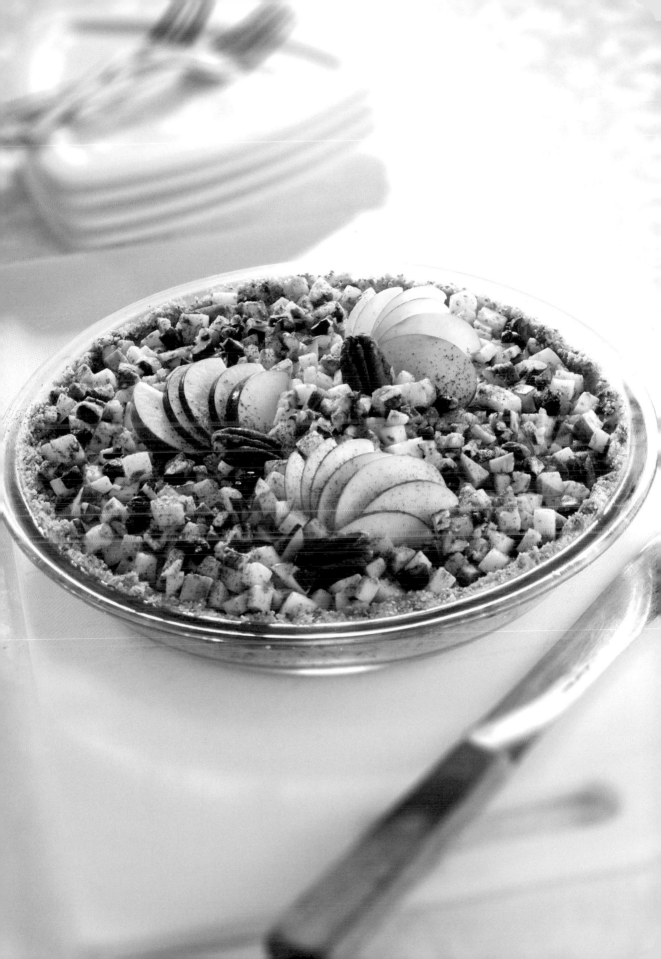

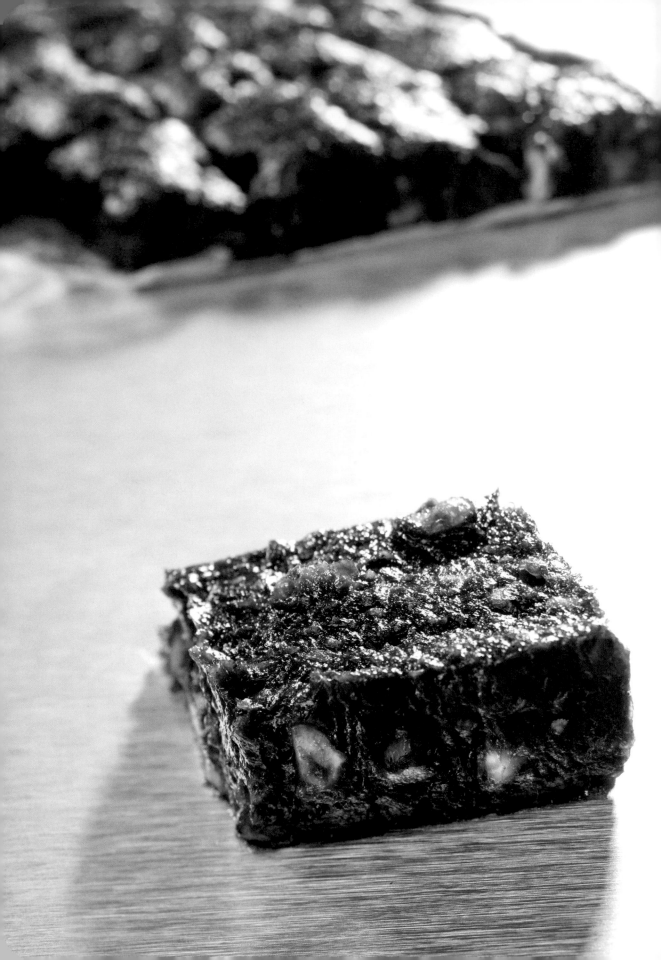

Melt-In-Your-Mouth Brownies

25 brownies • PREPARATION: 20 minutes • REFRIGERATION TIME: 2 hours

METHOD

In a food processor or with a whisk, combine all ingredients.

Line a 9-inch (23 cm) square dish with parchment paper. Place mixture in prepared dish and press with your hands to flatten it.

Refrigerate at least 2 hours. Cut into 25 squares.

INGREDIENTS

¼ cup (60 ml) honey or maple syrup

¼ cup (60 ml) cocoa powder, sifted

Pinch cayenne pepper

1 tsp ground cinnamon

2 ripe avocados, puréed

1 cup (250 ml) hazelnuts or other nuts, coarsely chopped

1 cup (250 ml) dates, chopped

**Nutrition Facts
Per brownie**

Amount	% Daily Value
Calories 100	
Fat 6 g	9%
Saturated 0.5 g	3%
+ Trans 0 g	
Polyunsaturated 0.5 g	
Omega-6 0.5 g	
Omega-3 0 g	
Monounsaturated 4 g	
Cholesterol 0 mg	0%
Sodium 2 mg	0%
Potassium 170 mg	5%
Carbohydrate 11 g	4%
Fiber 2 g	8%
Sugars 7 g	
Protein 1 g	
Vitamin A 3 RE	0%
Vitamin C 2 mg	2%
Calcium 19 mg	2%
Iron 0.5 mg	4%
Phosphorous 36 mg	4%

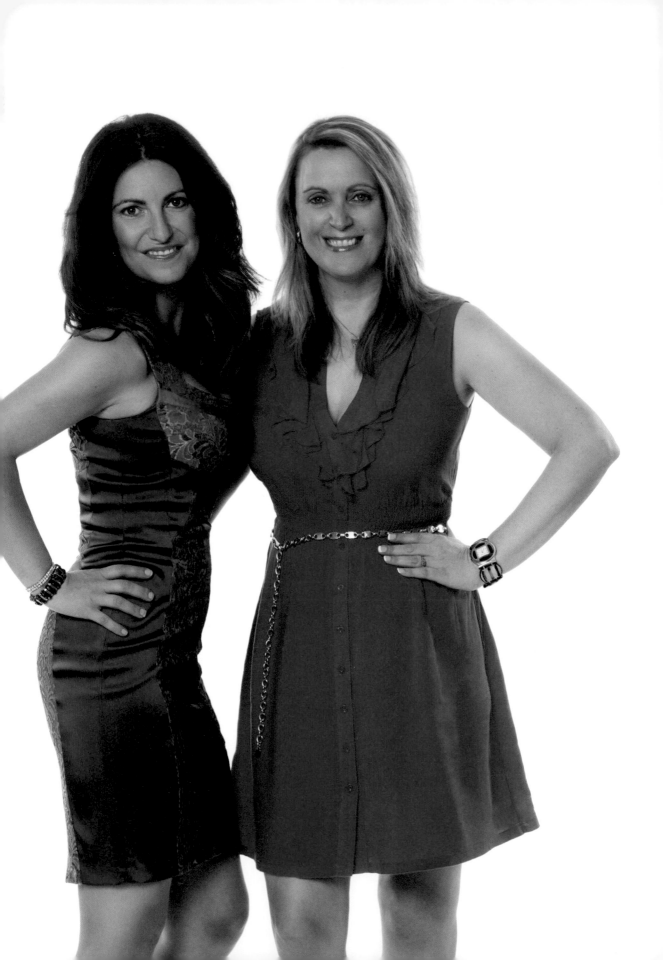

Elisabeth Cerqueira is co-president of NutriSimple, a network of over 45 private nutrition clinics in Quebec. She is also the coauthor of *Weight Loss* in the Know What to Eat series. She has a bachelor's degree in nutrition from McGill University. She is a registered dietitian and is a member of the Ordre professionnel des diététistes du Québec (Professional College of Dietitians of Quebec).

For over 15 years, Elisabeth has been teaching clients to eat by helping them increase the nutritional value of their food. She treats food imbalances that lead to obesity, diabetes, cholesterol, arthritis, anorexia and more. Her mission is to be her clients' partner in health. At the leading edge of scientific research, she and her team of nutritionists offer a simple nutritional program. Her empirical approach promotes a diet that helps clients get in peak shape. She is known for her passion for nutrition in medical circles and in the arts. She was a nutritionist to celebrities including actor Gerard Butler, in the movie *300*.

Elisabeth loves to cook with her three children and applies the advice offered at NutriSimple. She believes that eating well should be a simple pleasure. From a European background, she enjoys life's pleasures, including food.

elisabeth@nutrisimple.com
nutrisimple.com

Marise Charron graduated in nutrition from Laval University and has been a practicing registered dietitian for over 20 years. She is the author of a number of successful cookbooks and loves to share her knowledge of nutrition and cooking, two related areas that she is passionate about. Marise loves discovering and inventing new recipes and believes that eating well means savoring the moment.

In 1991, Marise founded Groupe Harmonie Santé to provide professional development to dietitians in private practice and promote discussion among health care professionals. In 2010, she teamed up with Elisabeth Cerqueira to create NutriSimple.

An entrepreneur at heart, she is also at the helm of Nutrition2C (nutrition2c.com), which offers a nutritional analysis and labelling service to companies, schools, restaurants and magazines. In 1998, the Ordre professionnel des diététistes duQuébec (Professional College of Dietitians of Quebec) recognized her work with the Annual Merit Award in Nutrition.

As a clinical dietitian, Marise loves the close relationship she develops with her clients, recommending healthy habits using an approach that respects body diversity.

marise@nutrisimple.com
nutrisimple.com

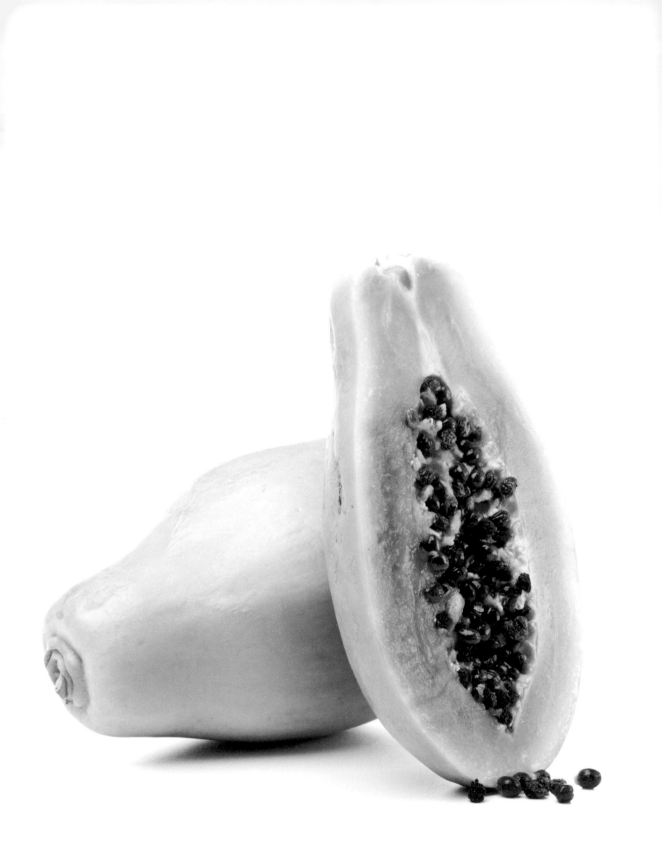

ACKNOWLEDGMENTS

We would like to thank our publishers for their trust, particularly Marc Alain, publisher of Modus Vivendi, and Isabelle Jodoin, our senior editor, who supported us throughout this project.

Thanks as well to copy editor Nolwenn Gouezel for her tips and suggestions, and graphic designers Émilie Houle and Gabrielle Lecomte for the wonderful layout. And, of course, a big thanks to photographer André Noël and food stylist Gabrielle Dalessandro.

A number of dietitians reviewed this book, for which we thank them, because their invaluable comments made it better. We are very grateful to them. So thank you to fellow dietitians. Audrey Cyr, Linda Montpetit, Josiane Lanthier, Marie-Hélène Carrier, Nadia Courchesne and Andréanne Martin.

We would also like to acknowledge the amazing help of our colleague Marlène Bouillon, dietitian and Ph.D. Thank you, Marlène, for your critical insight and eagle eye. We are fortunate to have crossed paths with you.

Thank you also to all of our clients who trust us during nutritional consultations.

Finally, we would also like to thank our raison d'êtres, the loves of our lives: our spouses, Pierre and Jack, who patiently supported us while we were writing this book, and our children, without whom life wouldn't be worth living. We love you all very much, and thank you for your patience.

Thank you in advance to all those who buy this book, who visit our website and who will share their experiences to help as many people as possible live pain-free.

RESOURCES
for Arthritis Sufferers

NORTH AMERICA
American College of Rheumatology
www.rheumatology.org

Office of Dietary Supplements, National Institutes of Health
www.ods.od.nih.gov

Arthritis Broadcast Network
www.arthritisbroadcastnetwork.org

JointHealth
www.jointhealth.org

Canadian Rheumatology Association
www.rheum.ca

The Arthritis Society
www.arthritis.ca

Public Health Agency of Canada
www.phac-aspc.gc.ca/cd-mc/arthritis-arthrite

EUROPE
National Rheumatoid Arthritis Society
www.nras.org.uk

AUSTRALIA
Arthritis Australia
www.arthritisaustralia.com.au

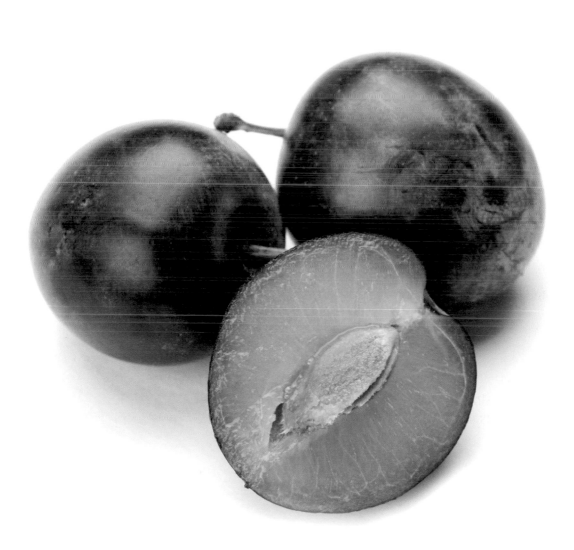

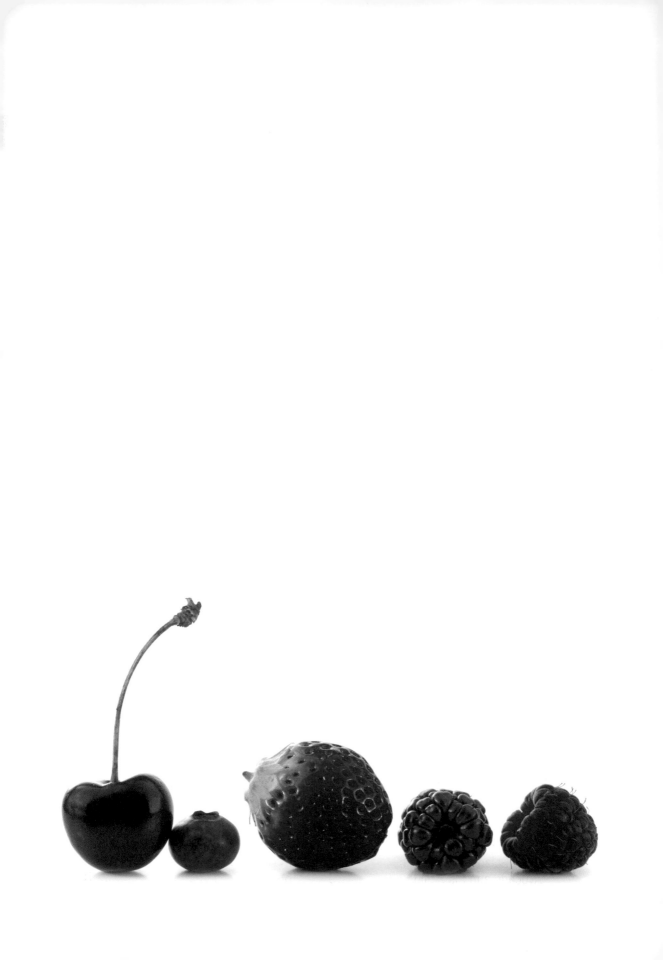

RECIPE Index

DRINKS

Anti-Inflammatory Smoothie 64

Anti-Inflammatory Water 60

Incredible Green Smoothies 62

Quick and Easy Smoothies 67

BREAKFASTS AND SWEET SNACKS

Berry Easy Pudding 74

Flourless, Bakeless
Anti-Inflammatory Balls 68

Healthy Truffles............................... 69

Morning Snack................................ 70

Pancakes with Pear and Cinnamon.... 72

APPETIZERS, SIDES AND SAVORY SNACKS

Buckwheat Flax Crackers 80

Delectable Veggie Pâté 76

Kale Chips...................................... 84

Healthy Hummus 82

Root Vegetable Pâté 79

SOUPS AND SALADS

Buckwheat Salad with Pomegranate
and Edamame 98

Fennel and Orange Salad 96

Gingery Carrot Soup 101

Gingery Sweet Potato Soup 89

Indian Salad 92

Italian Salad with Chickpeas
and Quinoa 102

Quick and Easy Kale Salad 86

Quinoa Apple Salad 108

Quinoa Pineapple Salad with
Turmeric Vinaigrette 104

Quinoa Salad with Cucumber,
Avocado and Pistachios................ 94

Summer Quinoa 106

Versatile Salad................................ 90

MAIN COURSES

Asian Tofu and Turkey Stir-Fry........ 114

Chicken with Mango Salsa.............. 126

Easy Peasy Indian Chicken 130

Fiesta Vegetable Frittata 124

Fish en Papillote 136

Fish Fillets with Fines Herbes 134

Indiana Salmon Cakes 116

Kale Stuffed with Poultry
and Basmati Rice....................... 141

Meatless Bolognese Sauce 143

Nut-Crusted Salmon 139

Rice Vermicelli with Pesto and Fish ... 111

Rice Vermicelli with Salmon
and Ginger................................. 132

Salmon Fillets with
Anti-Inflammatory Spices............. 112

Salmon with Avocado and
Citrus Salsa 129

Spring Rolls................................. 118

Turkey with Basil Pesto
and Cabbage............................. 122

Vegan Makis................................ 121

DESSERTS

Anti-Inflammatory Quinoa Drops...... 146

Flourless, Bakeless Cinnamon
Apple Crisp............................... 148

Summer Fruit Salad with
Chia Seeds 144

Surprising Melt-In-Your-Mouth
Brownies 151

KNOW WHAT TO EAT

A diet suited to your needs based on advice from expert dietitians

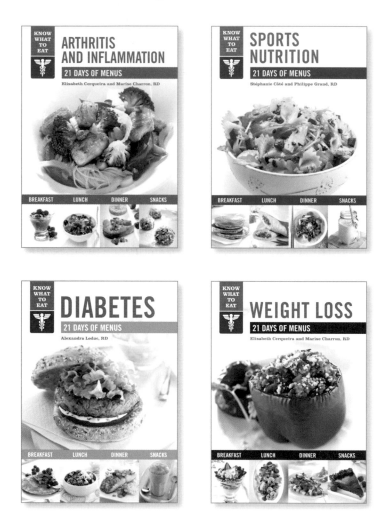

MODUSVIVENDIPUBLISHING.COM